Reprinted from Bibliographia Genetica XIX

ISBN 978-94-015-1684-6   ISBN 978-94-015-2827-6 (eBook)
DOI 10.1007/978-94-015-2827-6

Bibliographia Genetica XIX (1960): 1–86.

CYTOGENETICS OF RYE (*SECALE SPP.*)

by

S. K. JAIN[1])

Department of Genetics, University of California, Davis, California.

(*Received for publication February 16, 1959*)

CONTENTS

[1]) During the latter part of this study, the writer received an Agriculture Fellowship, 1958–59, of University of California which is gratefully acknowledged. He is also indebted to Prof. G. L. STEBBINS for providing the material and laboratory facilities, and for many helpful discussions.

INTRODUCTION

Rye first appeared rather late in the history of human civilization. The oldest archaeological records of rye date from the Hallstatt period in Silesia, Thuringia and Westfalia and from the Lacène period. After the pioneering work of N. I. VAVILOV on the origin of cultivated plants three broad classes came in recognition: wild, weedy and cultivated rye. As a crop, rye is most winterhardy of all cereals so that in Northern Europe its cultivation reaches beyond the Arctic circle in Finland. While Soviet Russia contributes most to the total world production, in Finland, Poland, Germany, Sweden, Netherlands and Belgium also its rank is high among grain crops. It is striking to note that for the past many years, research on practical agronomical and breeding problems has been quite active in these countries and currently attempts to improve rye are being made on modern lines. Some of the main problems in this field concern with the development of hybrid varieties, improvement of autotetraploid fertility, use of best pollination procedures to obtain highly self-fertile lines and the transfer of rye characters to wheat as such or in the form of amphiploid Triticales. In Russia, however, the Michurinist agrobiologists are primarily engaged in the study of interspecific conversions, branched ear types and nutritional methods of improving varieties, and perhaps this is one reason of only little having been known about rye genetics. As a material for cytological research, however, rye has been generally favoured and indeed such of its features as possibility of studying pachytene chromosomes, success of autotetraploidy and the occurrence of B-chromosomes are now well known.

During the past few years, interesting beginnings have been made on various aspects of rye cytogenetics. Previous reviews on the genus *Secale* include those of AASE (1935, 1946) dealing with the cytology of cereals, of O'MARA (1953) on the cytogenetics of *Triticale*, and of LAUBE and QUADT (1956) giving special attention to breeding aspects. The present paper therefore attempts to bring together important cyto-genetic information now available in this genus and it does not ad-mittedly pretend to be comprehensive, one important reason being the fact that original papers published in Russian, Japanese, etc. unfortu-nately could not be used. While the sections on cytology and genetics are somewhat detailed, those on systematics and origin of cultivated rye only briefly indicate the present status of our knowledge on them.

I. CYTOLOGY

1. Chromosome numbers

NEMEC (1910) was probably the first to record the chromosome counts in *Secale cereale*. He observed 18 chromosomes in endosperm cells. Two other reports, those of WESTIGATE (cited after STOLZE, 1925) and of SPILLMAN (cited after HECTOR, 1934), gave 12 as the somatic number. NAKAO (1911) on the other hand found n = 8 in the first metaphase plates of microsporogenesis. Following this appeared SAKAMURA'S (1918) count of 2n = 14 and later KIHARA (1924) who found some cells with n = 8 in plants having 2n = 14, tried to explain these discrepant counts on the basis of extra chromosomes. According to FERRAND (1923), ocasional nondisjunction of one the seven bivalents gave rise to plants with an extra pair whereas cells with even higher numbers could arise by fragmentation at some stage. Still the haploid number remained uncertain until a number of careful mitotic and meiotic counts along with the analyses of extra chromosomes, established 7 as the correct one (STOLZE, 1925; AASE and POWERS, 1926; THOMPSON, 1926; EMME, 1927; LEWITSKY, 1929, 1931; and others) and higher numbers of 8, 9, or 10 being for the strains carrying B-chomosomes (EMME, 1928; DARLINGTON, 1933; HASEGAWA, 1934; POPOFF, 1939; MÜNTZING, 1944, *et seq.*).

In many of these early papers, the material was not specifically mentioned and EMME (1928) criticizing this point, described her own materials carefully. She reported chromosome numbers in *S. fragile* M.B. (2n = 14, 16), in *S. africanum* Stapf. (2n = 15, 16) and in *S. cereale* var. *afghanicum* Vav. (2n = 16). Other reports of chromosome number in these related species of *cereale* rye include those of 2n = 14 in *S. ancestrale* (KOSTOFF *et al*, 1935), and 2n = 14, 16 in *S. montanum* (STAHLIN, 1929; KOSTOFF *et al*, 1935), in *S. fragile* (LEWITSKY, 1931), in *S. africanum* (GNOWS, cited after DARLINGTON and WYLIE, 1956), in *S. Kuprijanovii*(NAKAJIMA, 1954) and in *S. vavilovii* (NAKAJIMA, 1953 b). Two other species namely *anatolicum* and *dalmaticum* are considered to be ecotypes of *montanum* (STUTZ, 1957; also see Sec. III) Thus it appears that if we disregard the presence of accessories, all known species of this genus have seven pairs of chromosomes. DAR-LINGTON and WYLIE (1956) listed tetraploid rye separately perhaps in view of its almost complete reproductive isolation from diploid rye (Section ID). However in present paper, 14, and 28 will be considered as diploid and tetraploid numbers respectively.

2. *Cytological Techniques.*

Most rye workers in past used paraffin sectioning in their cytological investigations. In order to emphasize the importance of finding suitable pretreatments and methods of fixation and staining for a specific purpose, a few of them are reviewed below:

I) LEWITSKY (1931). Fix in a mixture of 5–10% formalin and 1% chromic acid (1 : 1). Stain with iron hematoxylin.

II) SHMARGON (1938). Fix in Lewitsky's strong Platinic-formalin soln. Stain with iron hematoxylin.

III) PATHAK (1940). Pretreat with 0.4% chloral hydrate; fix in Benda's fluid (without acetic acid); dehydrate by chloroform as usual and stain in iodine gentian-violet or light-green.

IV) LEVAN (1942). With or without cold treatment; fix in Navashin's or Lewitsky's fluid and stain with gentian-violet supplemented by Feulgen. Nucleolus staining by Bhaduri's light green.

V) TJIO and LEVAN (1950). Pretreat with 8-hydroxyquinoline (0.002 M/litre i.e. 0.29 gm.per litre of water) for 2–6 hours; transfer to stain-hydrochloric acid mixture (2% acetic-orcein, 9 parts and N HCl 1 part); warm to macerate and smear in a drop of acetic-orcein.

VI) MÜNTZING and his associates: Fix in chrome-acetic-formalin; stain with crystal violet. MÜNTZING (1951a) placed tetraploid material overnight at 0°C to shorten the chromosomes before fixing.

In the opinion of the present writer, the technique of TJIO and LEVAN, as modified by PRAKKEN and SWAMINATHAN (1951), is satisfactory for all work on roottip chromosomes. Feulgen squashing combined with a pretreatment with weak solutions of colchicine and paradichlorobenzene may also be found useful. For the study of meiotic chromosomes, simple aceto- or propionocarmine smears and also Feulgen method have been successfully used. To make permanent slides, this writer found the latter more convenient to be followed by vapor-chamber method of BRADLEY (1948).

3. Chromosome morphology

(a) Cytological maps. GOTOH (1924) first reported the measurements of somatic chromosomes in strains with 2n=14 and 2n=16 (i.e. with two accessory chromosomes) and found that total lengths of karyotype were nearly equal so that these extra chromosomes seemed to be directly derived by diminution of the original complement. EMME (1928) gave support to this from her studies in two other species, *S. montanum* and *S. africanum*. She pointed out, however, that such karyotype studies in a variety of materials would be most revealing in understanding the systematics and phylogeny of the genus.

Classical work by LEWITSKY (1929, 1931) further reported chromosome measurements and maps in a number of *cereale* strains and other species, with particular reference to arm-ratio and position of satellites. His criticism of EMME (1927, 1928) for her vague statements such as "in two cases satellites were found" or "constrictions in long chromosomes are of frequent occurrence" does seem valid although his own drawings are not too clear. In Table I, the results of the writer's own observations and those by LEWITSKY (1931), SHMARGON (1938a, b) and OINUMA (1953a, b) on root tip chromosomes are given to provide comparison and it will be apparent that except for LEWITSKY's, other data agree fairly well, the minor differences being partly attributable to the diversity of material used and the technique as well. Here it may be pointed out that in general, both the absolute measurements of individual chromosomes as well as their relative sizes can vary within fairly wide limits depending on several factors and hence allowance need be made in any such comparisons.

SHMARGON (1938 a, b; 1939) recorded measurements in terms of 'chromomere' number considering each one of them as being compounded from several pachytene chromomeres. For instance, according to this author, the nucleolar pair has approximately fifty pachytene chromomeres showing at mitosis as 11 compound 'chromomeres'. It is therefore obscure how these data can be interpreted in linear units. OINUMA's (1952, 1953 a, b) studies included several different strains and following his scheme of designating karyotype races based on positions of primary and secondary constrictions, a total of seven such races could be recognized. His analyses of two more strains, Korean 1 and 2, further established the value of karyotype study in work with B-chromosomes. The most common B-chromosome, the standard fragment (Section 1C), has been measured in several different strains and again the data seem to be approximately in agreement. From the reports of arm ratio in the extra chromosome, (1 : 4, HASEGAWA, 1934; 1 : 7. DARLINGTON, 1933; and terminal centromere, GOTOH, 1932), it would appear that different B-chromosomes were being studied.

LIMA-DE-FARIA (1948) worked out certain details of acetocarmine smear technique for studying pachytene chromosomes in rye and thanks to his painstaking researches, today a great deal is known about its karyotype as well as B-chromosomes. Table 1(b) gives a

TABLE I. Data on chromosome morphology in rye (*Secale cereale*).

(a) Root tip mitosis

Chr. No.	Measurements in μ		Total	Arm ratio approx.	Arm ratio given by		
	L.A.	R.A.			LEWITSKY (1931)	SHMARGON (1938a, b)	OINUMA (1953a, b)
I	5.4	4.7	10.1	1 : 1·1	1 : 5	1 : 2	1 : 1
II	4.9	4.8	9.7	1 : 1·0	1 : 1	1 : 1·5	1 : 1·5
III	4.6	4.1	8.7	1 : 1·1	1 : 5	1 : 2	1 : 1
IV	4.2	3.8	8.0	1 : 1·1	1 : 1	1 : 1	1 : 1
V	4.4	3.5	7.9	1 : 1·3	1 : 1	1 : 1	1 : 2
VI	5.0	2.9	7.9	1 : 1·7	1 : 7	1 : 1	1 : 1·5
VII*	4.8	2.7	7.5	1 : 1·8	1 : 2	1 : 1	1 : 1

(b) Pachytene of microsporogenesis (From LIMA-DE-FARIA, 1952b).

Chr. No.	Measurements in μ		R.A.	Total	Arm ratio	Knobs
	L.A.	SA				
I	37.0	3.4	50.4	90.7	1 : 1·4	both ends
II	39.6	2.9	45.8	88.3	1 : 1·2	right arm
III	33.9	3.2	45.3	82.3	1 : 1·3	both ends
IV	39.6	2.8	36.5	78.8	1 : 1·1	,,
V*	24.6	2.5	42.5	69.6	1 : 1·7	,,
VI	23.5	3.6	48.8	75.9	1 : 2·1	left arm
VII	21.8	2.9	58.4	83.2	1 : 1·7	,,

L.A. = Left arm.   R.A. = Right arm.   SA = centromere   * Nucleolar pair.

summary of Lima-de-Faria's (1952b) data on chromosome measurements. It is enlightening to note close agreement between mitotic and pachytene observations, with one notable exception of chromosome III (Table Ia) and VII according to Lima-de-Faria's data. To sum up, the chromosome complement of rye has its four or five largest pairs median or submedian, and others submedian to subterminal, the smallest pair being associated with the nucleolus and having a satellite. One or two more pairs of satellites sometimes appear in cold-treated material, or might be occasionally seen in some strains even without any treatment (For example, see Stutz, 1957; Riley and Chapman, 1958).

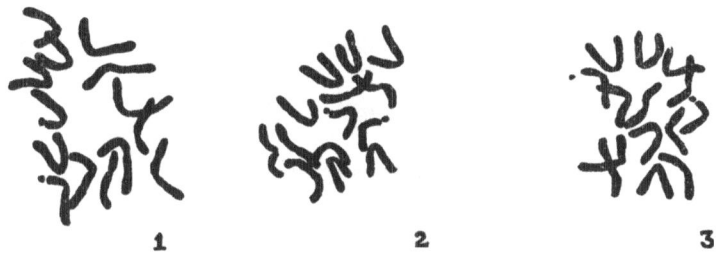

Figs. 1–3. Root tip chromosomes in *cereale*, *africanum* and *sylvestre* respectively. Note one satellited pair in each case and other general similarities of karyotype.

In figs. 1–3 are shown the typical somatic metaphase plates in three different species namely *cereale*, *africanum* and *sylvestre*. It appears that at least during mitosis their karyotypes do not show any differences. In our material no B-chromosomes could be found so far.

(b) Chromomeres and chromosome gradient.

Using pachytene stage of microsporogenesis, Lima-de-Faria (1948 *et seq.*) has constructed chromosome maps giving details of their chromomere pattern. These following features deserve special mention here. Firstly, all chromosomes including the standard fragment seem to exhibit a common basic pattern with only minor variations. Secondly, there exists a visible gradient on both sides of the centromere (Lima-de-Faria prefers the term kinetochore) with smaller chromomeres towards the chromosome ends up to the large knob-formations.

Thus it was assumed that size of a chromomere is a function of both the genotype and its position on the chromosome. Thirdly, at pachytene the presence of heterochromatic regions is not identifiable, there being no visible difference in their structural organization. A few such regions, however, have been inferred to be present terminally (for

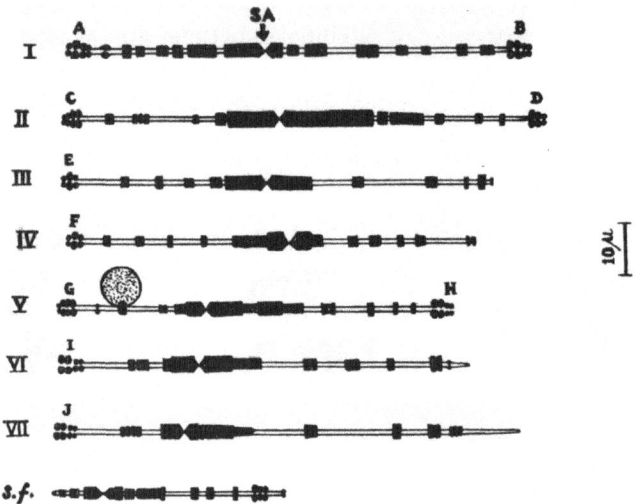

Fig. 4. A highly diagrammatic map of pachytene chromosomes in rye based on those given by LIMA-DE-FARIA (1952b) with all their chromomeric details. Note that here only relatively large chromomeres or chromatin blocks are shown which the present writer believes from his study as rather easily identifiable. (A–J, knob-formations; s.f., standard fragment; SA, centromere region).

instance, REES, 1955 a; and BOSE, 1956). Finally, certain chromomeres by virtue of their size and shape characteristics provide useful landmarks of the differential regions along a chromosome. Some chromomeres, for example, have fibrillae on them. LIMA-DE-FARIA (1952 a, b) found that except for III from IV and VI from VII, others can be easily identified. It is important to note here that PATHAK (1940) considered this very fact as an evidence of 5 being the basic number of rye so that in its complement secondary polyploidy was assumed, but this view has not found any support lately by many authors.

(c) The kinetochore structure and the satellites.

As opposed to the general consensus of opinion that centromere is merely a constriction (hence the term primary constriction), recently its structure has come to be known, again due to brilliant work by LIMA-DE-FARIA (1949, 1956). He showed that kinetochore too has chromomeric organization and accordingly three different zones were marked as an exterior zone, a central chromomeric zone and an interior zone, their respective properties being (a) connection with the arms, (b) active mobility and (c) special division cycle. Some evidence could be obtained from the study of a fragment with deleted kinetochore which had only a weakly stainable fibrilla pair and a pair of chromomeres, moved normally to the poles but was eliminated during the second meiotic division. These results clearly show the importance of studying the structure of kinetochore especially while dealing with the problem of chromosome duplication and movements.

It was mentioned earlier that a normal complement of rye has a pair of satellited chromosomes while two or more have also been recorded. LEVAN (1942) observed regularly one or two pairs of satellites in untreated material whereas after the low temperature treatments of somatic nuclei, three more pairs besides s_1 and s_2 showed satellite-like regions. Of these s_4 showed a clear achromatic segment in the middle of its longer arm which appears therefore to correspond to one in the amphibivalent observed by MÜNTZING and PRAKKEN (1941). LEVAN (1942) further pointed out that these regions differentiated mostly at the end of shorter arms, later confirmed by the studies of TJIO and LEVAN (1950) and of LIMA-DE-FARIA (1952b). These workers inferred the presence of heterochromatin in these localised regions so that following the hypothesis putforth by DARLINGTON and LACOUR (1940), this differentiation is a result of nucleic acid starvation while competing with the euchromatic regions. An alternative explanation can be based on their differences in the amount or type of coiling, as for instance, REES (1955 a) recorded certain cells in this inbred material showing uncoiled chromosome regions towards their ends.

Moreover, LIMA-DE-FARIA (1952 a, b) observed large chromomeres in terminal positions which he designates as knob-formations (Table 1b). Earlier, TJIO and LEVAN (1950) had counted as many as 20 knobs, both terminal and intercalary inclusive, in root tip nuclei during prophase but as they point out, these are heteropycnotic and might consist of some kind of heterochromatin. Thus all of them do not seem to be conspicuous at pachytene for one reason or another. Even the size of one of the knob-formations was found to vary among different strains from Sweden and Turkey (LIMA-DE-FARIA, 1952 b).

More recently, LIMA-DE-FARIA and SARVELLA (1958) have studied the structure of the terminal chromomere, the telomere or telochromomere. In rye, a telomere was shown to consist of at least 8 segments – 4 chromomeres and 4 fibrillae – all of them having the property of unipolarity which is a distinct property of this terminal structure. That how far these observations hold generality in terms of structure as well as function is difficult to say at this stage. Nonetheless, all the aforementioned features of a karyotype put together, can provide information the importance of which needs no overemphasis.

B. MEIOTIC STUDIES IN SPECIES

1. *General observations.*

In all species material that has been studied cytologically, in general, meiosis is found to be regular, seven bivalents (see Section C for meiotic study of B-chromosomes that are present in some strains only) being formed in nearly every cell at first prophase and metaphase. As shown in Table 2 below, only about 0–15% cells show the presence of two univalents with six bivalents thus giving a mean figure of 0.0–0.3 univalent per cell. However, there is considerable variation in respect with the relative proportions of ring and rod bivalents, or which is sometimes tantamount to chiasma frequency. Except for RILEY's (1956) data of *S. montanum*, other variation may be simply due to sampling errors, or minor environmental differences. It is significant to note that chiasma frequencies in different species seemed to vary characteristically and data recorded for variances between and within plants indicated correlations between mean chiasma frequency and variance (JAIN, unpub.).

The occasional anaphase irregularities included bridges, laggards or nondisjunctive tendency of a bivalent. EMME (1928) found two chromosomes in *montanum* to be held together continually during meiosis so that at II M, only six chromosomes seemed countable. Earlier,

FERRAND (1923) reported a rather high frequency of irregular divisions in *cereale* rye giving rise to cells with varying number of chromosomes which he postulated to be resulting from nondisjunction and also occasional fragmentation. Observations of STEBBINS and JAIN

TABLE 2. Summary of meiotic data in species.

Species	Reference	I M pairing (Mean per cell)			Xta/cell	% Irreg. I A cells
		Uni.	Rods	Rings		
cereale	SCHIEMANN & KRÜGER	—	—	7.0		
,,	PRICE	0.21	6.89		14.4	3.5
,,	RILEY	—	0.4	6.6		
,.	STEBBINS & JAIN	0.14	0.48	6.45	15.12	3.7
montanum	SCHIEMANN & KRÜGER	—	—	7.0		
,,	RILEY	0.32	2.04	4.8		
dalmaticum	,,	0.24	0.92	5.96		
africanum	SCHIEMANN & KRÜGER	—	1.0	6.0		2.7
,,	STEBBINS & JAIN	0.12	0.56	6.38	13.75	4.2
vavilovii	,,	0.29	0.93	5.80	13.52	8.4
,, (?)	NAKAJIMA	0.18	6.91			
sylvestre	STEBBINS & JAIN	0.04	0.62	6.36	14.15	1.8

(unpub.) showed the occurrence of about 5% irregular II anaphase cells and only 1.5–4.5% microspores having micronuclei. In following section will be reviewed similar observations in material from natural populations as well as inbred strains.

2. *Studies in population rye.*

MÜNTZING (1939) reviewed and discussed at length the published evidence on the occurrence of structural heterozygosity in natural populations and its correlations with breeding systems, levels of fertility and evolutionary forces at work in these populations. *Secale cereale* is an example of naturally cross-pollinated species having self-incompatibility in high or very high degrees. Investigations by MÜNT-

ZING (1939; 1945; 1946b), MÜNTZING and PRAKKEN (1941) and PUTT (1954) have established the presence of chromosomal aberrations (mutations, in the broad sense of the term) in its natural populations.

Among a total of 167 plants from two populations and derived either directly from the population or from respective progenies of open-pollinated individuals, MÜNTZING and PRAKKEN (1941) found regular meiosis in 98 plants only whereas others showed various types of irregularities. Inversions and segmental interchanges could be observed

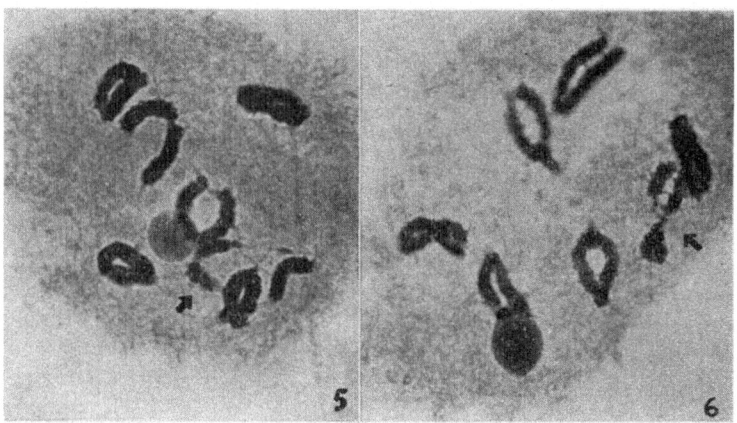

Figs. 5–6. Two PMC's at diakinesis of *S. vavilovii* plant having an irregular bivalent giving asynapsis. (From JAIN, 1959).

in respectively 5 and 6 plants and 2 others were found to be trisomics, one with accessory chromosomes and one diploid-tetraploid chimaera. Some of the frequent irregularities were such as nonconjunction during I M, or nondisjunction and fragmentation at I A. PUTT (1954) also recorded some irregularities in his material under study. Examples of only sporadic occurrence may include such aberrations as cytomixis with or without the presence of B-chromosomes (MÜNTZING and PRAKKEN, 1941), tripolar spindle (PUTT, 1954) and heteromorphic bivalent (JAIN, 1959). This peculiar bivalent occurred in only three of the *vavilovii* individuals grown during last winter and Figs. 5–6 show its appearance at diakinesis. I M pairing data were found to give a negative binomial distribution which might have some significance in explaining the origin and behaviour of this aberration (JAIN, 1958).

Perhaps of even greater interest are the cases of translocations and inversions. A detailed analysis by MÜNTZING and PRAKKEN (1941) showed that in three unrelated Stålråg plants having translocations, modal associations were IV + 5II or 2 IV + 3 II and that zigzag chains (i.e. with regular alternate disjunction) were preponderant. Further, it was suggested that only cryptic alterations might be involved since the multivalents were observed to be present in small sectors locally or even in single PMC's. For instance, one plant showed a trivalent in only a few cells. DARLINGTON (1933) also found an interchange to be present in a group of 8 cells which he considered to have originated by three successive divisions in a single initial cell. On the other hand, AKDIK and MÜNTZING (1949) recorded in two out of nine hybrids obtained from a cross between an Ecuadorian collection and. Swedish strain the presence of a quadrivalent so that it might indicate this translocation difference to be highly frequent. Here the homozygotes had to be crossed in order to detect the translocation. Similarly PUTT (1954) studied crosses between different lines of Emerald variety to note the occurrence of many translocation heterozygotes. Evidence for a difference of two translocations giving a ring-or chain-of-six chromosomes at diakinesis and metaphase I in the hybrids between members of *cereale*- group (includes *cereale* and *sylvestre*) and *montanum*-group(includes *montanum, africanum* and *vavilovii* among the better known species) is presented in a later section on interspecific hybridization. Some authors (viz. RILEY, 1956) believe that relative frequency of various chromosomal aberrations will be still higher in plants derived from unselected material rather than one maintained already for several years at research stations for study. No data seem to be available as yet on the natural incidence of translocation heterozygotes within or between different species growing together. A low frequency of dicentric bridges with fragments was observed at I A in a few cases (MÜNTZING and PRAKKEN, 1941) that seemed to suggest inversion segment as being only a small one. Some preliminary evidence for the presence of deficiencies and duplications in certain rye populations may be found in papers of MÜNTZING (1945), LIMA-DE-FARIA (1952b) and STUTZ (1957). Population analyses showing the distribution of B-chromosomes are mentioned elsewhere in this review (Section C 1). MÜNTZING (1946b) demonstrated that invariably all populations studied by him were genotypically different in respect with the presence of partial sterility (or 'Schartigkeit') and its variation.

3. Inbred rye.

LAMM (1936) initiated cytological study of inbred rye using *cereale* material inbred earlier by NILSSON-EHLE for 8 generations and found it to have pronounced meiotic disturbances and other differences such as lower chiasma frequency (1.06–2.41 per biv.) than in corresponding population rye (2.11–2.51 Xta per biv.). MATHER and LAMM (1935) had earlier shown that occurrence of univalents was inversely correlated with chiasma frequency and indeed LAMM'S (1936) observations confirmed it well. A careful analysis designed to show that the nucleolar (i.e. SAT-pair in this case) chromosomes could be present as univalents or as rod-or ring-bivalent, further suggested that lowered pairing tendency was not confined to any specific chromosome pairs. The univalents behaved typically, that is, they often divided and appeared as micronuclei in pollen grains, or at times as microcytes (REES, 1955a). Besides, other kinds of aberrations occasionally occurred such as cells with higher chromosome numbers (probably as a results of syndiploidy), unclean first anaphase separation, inversion or translocation configurations and chromosome breakage spontaneously. Double chromatid bridges with 2 fragments originated probably by double crossing-over and LAMM (1936) recorded also the chromosome contraction to have been reduced. Studies of AGEEW (1929) and KAKHIDZE (1939) on certain inbred Russian rye, in general, agree with the aforementioned results. MÜNTZING and AKDIK (1948b) reported their data on chromosome pairing during the first three inbreeding generations to show that in the first, there was no significant effect of inbreeding on meiotic behaviour; in second, very marked deterioration in amount of pairing; and in third again this had improved. They further observed a positive correlation within generations between chiasma frequency and plant vigour (measured in terms of plant height).

During his study of the effects of inbreeding (enforced self-fertilization) in Petkus rye for six generations (S_0 — S_5), SYBENGA (1958) observed, in general, strong effects on most of the characters under observation. The bulk of his data are summarily presented in Figure 7 below. Thus it can be seen how different characters responded with

varying amount and rate. Seed set(ss) after selfing gave a rapid increase only after S_1, seed set after free pollination (sf) a slight decrease
and percent pollen fertility a marked decline. SYBENGA was careful to

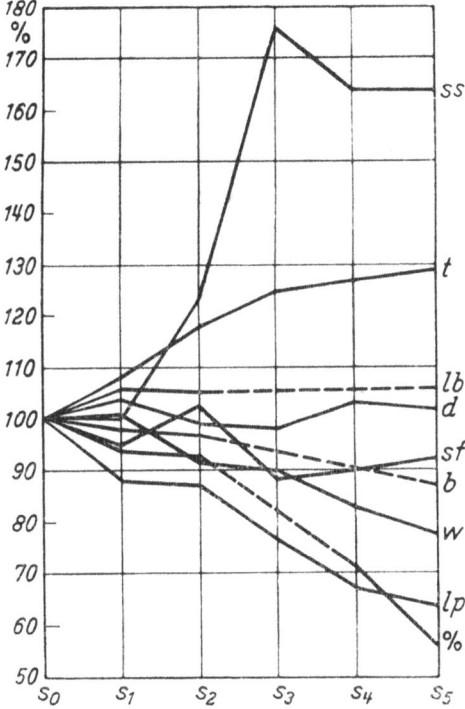

Fig. 7. Inbreeding curves. Generation averages
expressed in percent of S_0. *ss* seedset after selfing;
t number of tillers per plant; *lb* length of bivalents
at M I; *d* diameter of stem; *sf* seedset after free
pollination; *b* bound chromosome arms per cell;
w plant weight; *lp* plant height; % *fp* percent fertile
pollen. — — — data lacking for some generations
(From SYBENGA, 1958).

note various factors such as year effect, involuntary selection during
the inbreeding process or loss of chiasmata during metaphase by terminalization, that might disturb these results.

In their study of inbred rye, KATTERMANN (1939) and later PRAKKEN
and MÜNTZING (1942) observed an interesting phenomenon of socalled

T-ends, or "mobile chromosome ends", in which a chromosome pair seems to be having terminal 'centromere'. In a majority of cases such a neocentric activity was found to be arising in the shorter arm which then stretch and turn to the spindle poles. ÖSTERGREN and PRAKKEN (1946) also established the fact that true centromere was in submedian position and these T-ends might be having some properties simulating its behaviour during movement while they lacked the ability of holding together two sister chromatids from diplotene upto metaphase II. The number of pairs with such ends were found to be different among various materials (PRAKKEN and MÜNTZING, 0–6 pairs; REES, 1955a, 0–5 pairs). According to LIMA-DE-FARIA (1949, 1952b), this property might be correlated with the structural differentiation of a chromosome pair and the functioning of its centromere. Recently he has developed a concept based on chemical reasons of such a 'shift' in centromeric function.

The occurrence of certain premeiotic errors as inferred from the observations of MÜNTZING and AKDIK (1948b) and REES (1955a, b, 1957) represents another interesting feature in inbred rye. REES had derived two highly inbred lines from Stålråg (P2 and P5) of which P5 showed in about 1% of PMC's a variable number of extra fragments or entire chromosomes, some of them being initially somewhat retarded in division and the resulting micronuclei also behaved in varied ways that he considered to be due to certain cytoplasmic gradient differences. The cross between the lines P2 and P5 gave in F_1 and F_2 complete or nearly complete absence of premeiotic errors while in F_4 and F_5 again upto 8–9% PMC's showed them. It therefore suggests that this characteristic tendency is controlled genotypically and that inbreeding causes some unbalance thereby affecting its expressivity (REES, 1957). Similarly, data for chiasma frequency were as follows: average per cell in parental lines, 2.01 and 1.60; in F_1, F_2 and F_3, 2.25, 1.9, 1.7 respectively. In the same cross were found these other structural aberrations, namely (a) the appearance of uncoiled chromosomes (in about 1% PMC's), (b) anaphase bridges without fragments (in 16% cells) originating due to errors in splitting or stickiness near the chromosome ends, (c) anaphase bridges with fragments (about 20–50% cells in certain sublines) and (d) occasional ones like coenocytic nuclear groups, bivalent interlocking and spontaneous chromosome breakage. REES and THOMPSON (1955) observed in another inbred line P13 a lower terminalization coefficient and frequent breakages and REES (1955b) pointed out mutations or residual heterozygosity as possible causes. Earlier, LEITH and SHANDS (1938) in fact obtained evidence of residual heterozygosity being present in certain American inbreds. For many of these cytological aberrations mentioned above a genotypic control has been inferred.

4. Genotypic control of chromosome behaviour.

MÜNTZING and AKDIK (1948b) and more specifically REES (1955a) suggested that response to selection or the presence of a positive parent-offspring correlation should provide evidence of a genotypic control of chromosome behaviour. REES (1955 a,b) has convincingly shown that in rye the average plant chiasma frequency is genotypically controlled and also that the genotype influences the amount of non-heritable variation between PMC's within a plant. Furthermore, data of REES and THOMPSON (1956, 1957) indicate that even the response to varying environment depends on the genotype as for instance, they found this response to be in general greater in the inbred lines. These findings have an important place in our understanding of the mechanism of recombination as such and the operation of such genotypic factors as found in rye suggest that a relative uniformity among the gametes in respect with recombination might be an adaptive feature. As would be expected from above, REES (1957) found that the differences between families within F_3, F_4 and F_5 of an intravarietal cross were also genotypically controlled.

LAMM (1936) made the important observation that inbred rye had lower chiasma averages but higher terminalization coefficient which he explained on the basis of increased homology being an indirect cause of more terminalization. REES (1955a) however showed again from his data from within and between lines that the latter included genetic differences whereas variance for terminalization within lines may have resulted from mutations, or intense selection against homozygotes, or both. However, this cautions against any tacit assumption that lower chiasma frequency of inbreds indicates less recombination potential in them, if as in present example, this is accompanied simply by greater terminalization coefficient values.

Next, few instances of genotypically-controlled meristic characters might be briefly considered. MÜNTZING and PRAKKEN (1941) observed

a marked deficiency of translocation heterozygotes among the progenies raised from population samples. THOMPSON and REES (1956)
found two different interchange heterozygotes among their inbred
families of rye and of these one possessed selective advantage over the
two homozygotes, that was attributed to genetic balance factors.
By studying the variances in several successive generations,
THOMPSON (1956) established that the frequency of disjunctional
separation of rings or chains at anaphase I was under some kind of
genotypic control. Data of LAWRENCE (1958) on the relative disjunctional frequency from F_1 to F_6 are enlightening. Figure 8 shows
graphically the increase in both cases and according to LAWRENCE
(1958) it was an indirect result of selection within families for high
self-fertility since he observed not all plants giving the same amount
of seed. In a cross between two inbred lines, REES (1957) found that
certain new variants were arising through recombination between two
independently inherited characters, chiasma frequency and a structural aberration from premeiotic error. The occurrence of chimaeral
tissues for the latter he assumed to be genotypically determined.
Besides, the T-ends phenomenon (PRAKKEN and MÜNTZING, (1942;
REES, 1955a), chromosome size differences (PUTT, (1954) and occurrence of socalled P-bivalents (REES, 1955a) are also suggestive of a genotypic control of chromosome behaviour. Another interesting example
of probably genotypic control was given by MÜNTZING and AKDIK
(1948b) who considered weak staining of nuclear material (presumably
due to nucleic acid deficiency, according to them) to be associated with
other manifestations of inbreeding deterioration. A monogenic, recessive case of desynapsis was reported by PRAKKEN (1943) among the
inbred material and it might follow that such factors governing
chromosome behaviour accumulate in allogamous rye populations,
their numbers perhaps being inversely proportional to those for self-
sterility.

However, inbreeding effects on self-sterility character have been
studied by several authors (AGEEW, 1929; BREWBAKER, 1926; PETER-
SON, 1934; MENGERSEN, 1951; KRANZ, 1957). Their results are summarized later in a section on inheritance of self-sterility but here it may
be noted that in rye self-sterility is not too rigid so that attempts to
derive highly self-fertile lines have met with success. In fact, LUND-
QVIST (1958) has recently shown that homozygosity for certain chromo-

some regions he studied did not have deleterious effect on growth vigor or fertility of plants.

As to the explanation for inbreeding depression, an important although controversial paper was published by HERIBERT-NILSSON (1937) in rye. According to his new 'plasmon theory', the inbreeding effects are based on the plasmatic relationship between the parents and

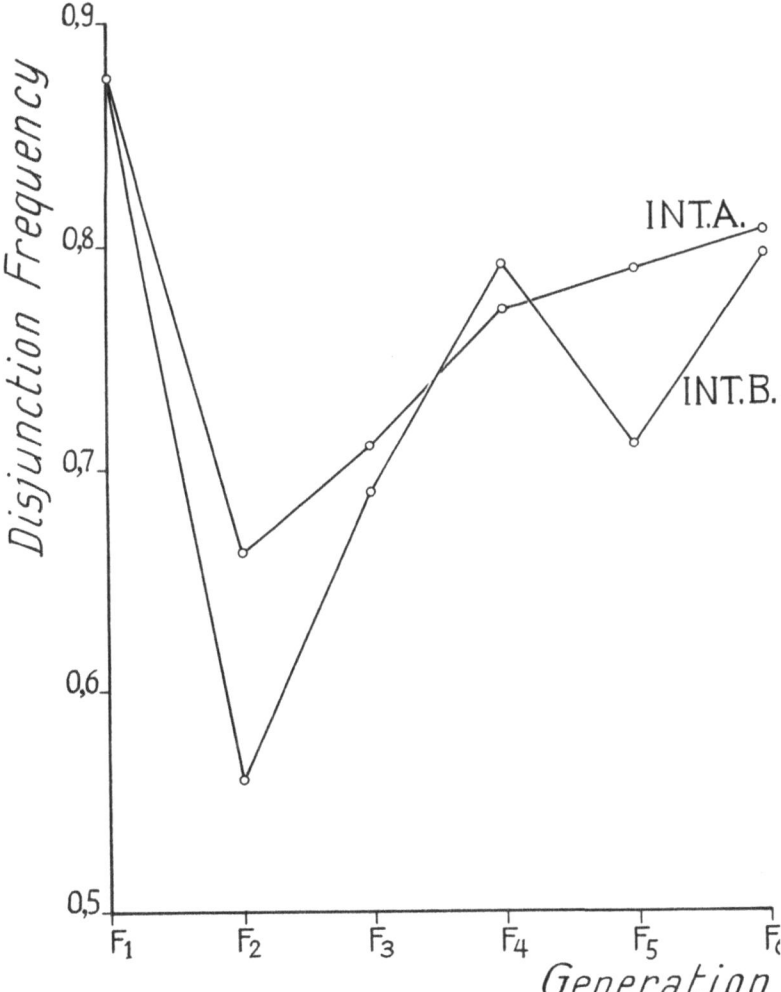

offsprings rather than any linked dominant gene interactions, or physiological reasons. So that more diverse the origin of plasma, less marked would be inbreeding decline which he claimed to have demonstrated using crosses with various grades of inbreeding. MÜNTZING and PRAKKEN (1941) were also inclined to admit some plasmatic cause as accounting for cytological aberrations that they had found in certain populations, SENGBUSCH (1940b) and NURNBERG-KRÜGER (1947, 1951), however, undertook some experiments to test the validity of plasmon theory as applied to explain the differences in inbreeding tolerance of rye and maize. The initial material of NURNBERG-KRÜGER comprised of a random group of 250 plants of Petkus rye and biometrical analyses of élite lines alongwith the pair-crosses established that rye was no exception to theory of inbreeding as developed for maize. In fact, a number of parallel studies on heterosis in rye are on record in literature (MAYER, 1944; FERWERDA, 1948, 1951; HAGBERG, 1952; MÜNTZING, 1954b; and many others reviewed in an excellent paper by LAUBE and QUADT, 1956). Further, MENGERSEN (1951) and MENGERSEN and SCHNELL (1956) point out several genetic implications of the practical aspects of heterosis common to rye and maize .

C. ACCESSORY OR B-CHROMOSOMES

1. Occurrence.

In a preceding section it was pointed out that a host of early workers recorded plants with 16 and even higher chromosome numbers in the natural populations of rye species. Some strains as those originating in Japan (KIHARA, 1924; GOTOH, 1924; BELLING, 1925; HASEGAWA, 1934), Russia (FERRAND, 1923; STOLZE, 1925; EMME, 1927; LEWITSKY, 1931; LEWITSKY et al, 1932), Bulgaria (POPOFF, 1939), Sweden (MÜNTZING, 1941, and later), Afghanistan and Turkey (MÜNTZING, 1950) and in Korea (OINUMA, 1953b; MÜNTZING, 1957) merit special mention here. A survey based on these studies will clearly show that the occurrence of B-chromosomes is relatively more common among the primitive strains and more so among those of Asiatic origin than of Europe. Some evidence for this is available from the work of MÜNTZING (1950) who analysed a few collections from various parts of Anatolia, one of the two centers of origin of cultivated rye that were suggested by the great pioneer N.I. VAVILOV – for the presence of B-chromosomes. His investigations on seven different strains from Korea gave similarly a wide range of frequencies, as for example, populations from Yonkii and Booyou regions had on an average 89.5–91.5% plants with B-chromosomes while the strain Seoul No. 2 gave the corresponding figure as 19.4% (MÜNTZING, 1957). Also, he found commercial strains almost devoid of the presence of B-chromosomes (MÜNTZING, 1954a).

Thus it would seem fairly obvious that a thorough and systematic study of their geographical distribution is needed in order to establish this probable correlation between the mode of occurrence of these accessory chromosomes and the ancestral route of spread of rye from its centers of origin. An important point should be made in this connection that although the socalled standard fragment type has been found to be very common, there are several others as well so that their structure, origin, homology with each other and so on should be kept in view.

2. Pachytene studies of B-chromosomes.

In course of their preliminary work, MÜNTZING and LIMA-DE-FARIA, 1949) were able to distinguish the standard fragment from a few other types of B-chromosomes (or, to use their term, extra fragments) by certain peculiarities in their meiotic behaviour. Subsequently the pachytene analysis enabled the identification of six different types, namely the standard fragment, the two telocentrics and the two corresponding isofragments and a deficiency fragment (See Fig. below). A brief description of each one follows.

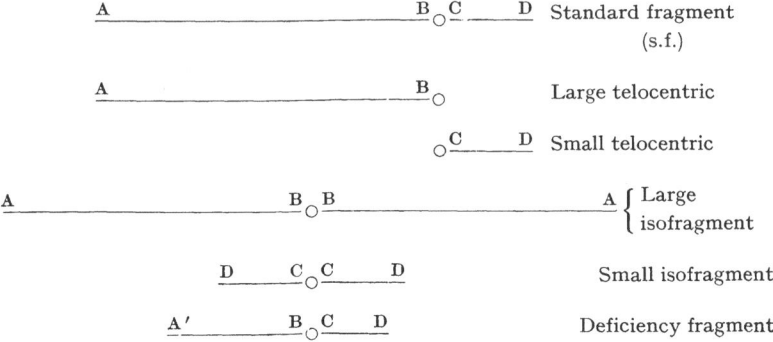

(a) Standard fragment. LEWITSKY (1931) and HASEGAWA (1934) had noted some of its morphological features in the cells of roottips and pollen grains respectively. The short arm is only about $\frac{1}{5}$th of total length and distally ends in a more or less oval head. During pachytene it measured about half as long as the shortest chromosome of the main complement (LIMA-DE-FARIA, 1948). MÜNTZING (1945) had recorded the length of standard fragment in somatic plates of two Swedish varieties (Östgota Gråråg and Vasa II) which gave 3.9μ and 4.4μ as respective figures and for the arm ratio 1 : 3.9 and 1 :4.5 approximately (MÜNTZING and LIMA-DE-FARIA, 1949). However the data were not sufficient in this case to establish an intervarietal difference statistically (LIMA-DE-FARIA, 1948). Some structural details are nevertheless of considerable interest and therefore will be mentioned next.

At the distal end of the longer arm there is a conspicuous knob and along the entire length three deeply stained and two other weakly stained regions were observed (LIMA-DE-FARIA, 1948; see also Fig. 4). Unlike the members of normal, or so to speak, A-complement that carry knobs only in terminal position, the standard fragment has its knob between those weakly stained regions. Besides, the chrommeres adjacent to its kinetochore are small and the gradient so marked in chromosomes of normal complement seems to be replaced by seriation of alternating large and small chromomeres (Fig. 4). MÜNTZING and LIMA-DE-FARIA (1949) also observed a slight difference in the size of 'appendage' distal to its knob among the plants of same two Swedish strains which could partly account for the data given by MÜNTZING (1945b). It is likely that these strains may show more such differences in their karyotype.

(b) Telocentrics and isofragments. MÜNTZING (1944) found from his study of microsporogenesis in Östgota Gråråg plants with 2n = 14 + one standard fragment that this extra unpaired fragment was cytologically unstable and gave rise occasionally to several new derivatives. For instance, simply by misdivision of its centromere (this happens when the centromere is split in transverse plane instead of longitudinal with respect to the chromosome linearity) two telocentrics arise corresponding to its arms. Pachytene study later confirmed this explanation as the chromomeric patterns of the standard fragment and two telocentrics together were found to be identical. Investigations on these telocentric fragments have provided excellent opportunity to follow the structural organization of the centromere. However these telocentrics are even more unstable, as would be expected from the fact that their fractured centromeres occupy a terminal position. SWANSON (1957) believes that one unequivocal case of telocentric chromosomes occurring in nature might be that of certain Protozoan species which represent special case as there are long centrioles associating with centromeres. However, in rye two isochromosomes originated apparently as a result of nondisjunctional division of the telocentrics, one being nearly five times larger than other. This could be confirmed again by pachytene analysis of their chromomeric makeup and other similar details (MÜNTZING and LIMA-DE-FARIA, 1949, 1953).

(c) Deficiency fragment (d.f.). MÜNTZING (1948b) observed another type of fragment which he formerly considered as to have derived by deletion of about half the longer arm of standard fragment. The actual measurements in the original plant and its progeny were 1.77μ and 1.98μ respectively, with a rather wide range of 1.56 to 2.20μ. To explain this variation MÜNTZING (1948b) assumed that such new derivatives were perhaps more influenced by certain mechanical variables acting during meiosis. Studies at pachytene showed that this fragment had in fact resulted from a terminal deficiency in the long arm of standard fragment (LIMA-DEFARIA, 1955a; MÜNTZING and LIMA-DE-FARIA 1952).

3. Meiotic studies.

As would be expected from the knowledge of the structure of these three different categories among B-chromosomes just mentioned, the meiotic behaviour and especially synapsis and disjunction that are of direct interest to us here, have been shown to differ among them. The standard fragment when present in two's per individual plant shows variable degrees of synapsis (with a fairly wide range). From his comparative study in two Swedish varieties (Östgota Gråråg and Vasa II), MÜNTZING (1945b) found that average frequencies of cells with two unpaired standard fragments were 61.8% (range 45–86%) and 11.1% (range 2–30%) respectively. DARLINGTON (1933)suggested that this frequency is predictable with fair accuracy if these three conditions, namely the chiasma frequency of A-complement, the relative length of fragment and its homology with other chromosomes, were known.

Thus the observed differences in varieties in this respect could be due
to either genotypic, or purely structural reasons. Some evidence of
genotypic control was actually obtained by MÜNTZING and LIMA-DE-
FARIA (1949) who found that there was equally good pairing between
standard fragments at the pachytene stage in both varieties. It is
significant to note that in plants with a single standard fragment and
so also those with two or more, MÜNTZING (1944) did not find them to
be paired with any chromosome of the normal complement which indicates lack of homology among this extra chromosome and others.
However, as was pointed out by him, critical evidence for this nonho-
mology should be better obtained by studying the haploids having a
standard fragment. Moreover, in all this work it is necessary to identify
properly the type of extra chromosomes present. For instance, GOTOH
(1924) and FETISSOV (1939) observed no pairing in their material
while DARLINGTON (1933), HASEGAWA (1934), YAKUWA (1944) and
others reported almost complete pairing. NAKAJIMA (1954c) recorded
the trivalent formation occasionally in this material with $2n = 19$.
Apparently, these workers might have been studying other types of
fragment chromosomes than the standard fragment.

In plants having large isofragments, MÜNTZING (1944) observed at
first metaphase two types of configurations: a rodshaped and large,
bent fragment with a visible median constriction, and a closed ring
type where presumably the two arms of an isochromosome were paired.
As many as 17% cells showed this latter configuration in all three plants
studied. In plants of variety Östgota Gråråg he (1951) later reported
about 26.3% cells with isobivalent formation which shows a reduction
of nearly 10% in comparison with the plants having standard fragments. MÜNTZING (1951b) was also able to demonstrate that pairing
in two isofragments of same cell is independent and that occasionally
a quadruple chiasma also formed.

On the other hand, the figures for the amount of pairing between
two small isofragments are much lower as for instance, MÜNTZING and
LIMA-DE-FARIA (1953) found only about 3% cells of a total of 200
examined having isofragments paired beyond doubt; a small percentage of those cells were doubtful cases. Further, it could be established
that this marked reduction in amount of pairing was due to their
small size because at pachytene and diplotene as many as 66% cells
showed pairing but without any visible chiasmata. A few cases of

pseudotetravalents or threearmed configurations were also recorded. (MÜNTZING and LIMA-DE-FARIA, 1953). The deficiency fragment is also very unstable and MÜNTZING (1948b) noted that in some cases it got eliminated from the sporogenous tissues while the somatic cells might show it to be present. Besides, he found that two deficiency fragments remained unpaired in all the cells he studied.

Data on their transmission, that is the relative frequencies in successive generations, are still more interesting. A series of experiments with plants having none, 1, 2 or higher numbers of B-chromosomes have shown that in the progenies of crosses among them most individuals had B-chromosomes in frequencies of even order, i.e. 2, 4, and so on. GOTOH (1924) crossed plants with 2n = 14 and 2n = 16 and in the hybrid progeny he found no plant with 2n = 15 and so also LEWITSKY *et al* (1932) obtained from the cross 2n = 18 × 2n = 18 plants with 2n = 16, 18 and 20. Another interesting feature of transmission is a tendency of numerical increase in succeeding generations. For instance, YAKUWA (1944) obtained the following data:

Cross	Number of B-chromosomes present in parents						
	0 × 2	2 × 0	0 × 3	0 × 4	4 × 0	2 × 2	4 × 4
Mean No. of B-chr. in progeny	1.4	1.5	1.75	3.5	2.8	3.8	7.0

It is apparent that these figures exceed significantly the expected ones in each case. The rate of this numerical rise in their occurrence may differ from one variety to another. MÜNTZING'S (1949) data from a study of two different varieties and in two consecutive years may be cited in support. He found in the progenies of a cross (0 × 2) i.e. between 2n = 14 and 2n = 16 plants, that the progeny mean figures were 3.58 and 3.38 for Östgota Gråråg and correspondingly 2.19 and 2.12 for Vasa II. One may also note that in this case the frequencies seem to have slightly decreased in the second year. To explain this one would probably have to assume that here an optimum was reached very rapidly so that in the period following this rise the genotype would be gradually adjusting the frequency of B-chromosomes to a level normally maintained. Using 15 different varieties MÜNTZING (1949) found for the same cross a range of 2.12 to 3.58

as progeny means and thence it would seem very interesting to study in greater detail the levels of optimum B-chromosome frequency in them and the nature of genetic mechanism that determines these properties.

The abovementioned features of transmission have been very well explained by the property of directional nondisjunction taking place during the maturation division of the gametes. HASEGAWA (1934) first observed in rye that during first pollen mitosis, the two daughter fragments at anaphase behaved irregularly and often reached the pole, or poles, later than others. Frequently both moved to the same pole (nondisjunction), and for some reason, more often to be included in the generative nucleus. Similar studies later with different B-chromosomes showed that the cause of nondisjunction lay not in any defect of the kinetochore but in some segment having stickiness or slower reduplication and since it was found that while large isofragment underwent nondisjunction like the standard fragment, the small one did not. MÜNTZING (1946a, and later) assumed this special segment to be located in the longer arm of standard fragment. Furthermore, the deficiency fragment does not also undergo nondisjunction so that the deficient knob might be the seat of this property. MÜNTZING (1945b) and HÅKANSSON (1948) obtained definite evidence of nondisjunction on the female side as well which is rather uncommon in many other genera having B-chromosomes (see BOSEMARK, 1957, for a review). In rye, although there does not seem direct evidence to be on record, from the data on progeny means it appears that the pollen having B-chromosomes preferentially fertilize the egg nuclei that too have them present until some upper limit was attained.

4. Phenotypic effects.

In general, the presence of B-chromosomes in a plant could not be ascertained from its phenotype alone. Nevertheless, there have been made few careful attempts to find out whether any such manifestation, subtle enough to have escaped notice, was present. A painstaking study was that by MÜNTZING and AKDIK (1948a) who measured the length of stomata for a total of 52 plants obtained from the crosses 2s.f. × 2s.f. and 2 l.isof. × 2 l.isof. Although their data seem to be heterogeneous, yet in plants with 2 and with 4 standard fragments about 5% and 12% increase in their stomatal lengths respectively was evident. Results with isofragments were also of the same order.

That B-chromosomes have some effect on meiosis and fertility of the 'carrier' individuals has been severally noted. FETISSOV (1939) recorded asynaptic tendency resulting in an extreme case the complete failure of pairing giving 16 univalents. However, MÜNTZING and PRAKKEN (1941) found much less severe effects and in their material (2n = 14 plus 2 s.f.) only about 5% cells were showing univalents (2 to 4). MÜNTZING (1946a, 1948b) was further able to show that the pollen mother cells with deficiency fragment were slightly retarded in developmental rate and likewise the pollen grains. HÅKANSSON (1957), on the other hand, observed that in plants with even 8 accessory chromosomes meiosis was fairly regular except that these accessories often gave only 2–4 bivalents, the univalents usually dividing at first anaphase. Nevertheless he found the first pollen or egg mitosis to be irregular resulting in lower fertility. Earlier POPOFF (1939) had concluded that the presence of B-chromosomes was always associated with such disturbances in fertility. MÜNTZING (1943c) also established this fact by showing an approximate but direct correlation between the number of B-chromosomes present and the failure of pollinations. He points out that the detrimental effects on vegetative characters such as culm height, plant height or kernel weight, are often conspicuous when as many as four B-chromosomes are present.

From above it appears that B-chromosomes are not as much genetically active as other chromosomes so that GOTOH's (1924) assumption would be discredited and similarly the approach by EMME (1928) to locating factors for rachis fragility on extra chromosomes. The question as to whether the B-chromosomes of rye are heterochromatic (now, whether heterochromatin is genetically inert appears itself to be problematic in view of many recent findings) is not yet settled. Earlier MÜNTZING (1943c, 1944) and LIMA-DE-FARIA (1948) had found no evidence of heteropycnosis in these chromosomes. At pachytene, however, LIMA-DE-FARIA (1952b) could show that the number and dimensions of positively and negatively heteropycnotic regions were greater in the case of the standard fragment than in A-chromosomes. It is therefore likely that B-chromosomes of rye represent an intermediate situation as suggested by LIMA-DE-FARIA (1952b).

5. Mode of origin and significance.

The issue about the possible mode of origin of B-chromosomes has in past given rise to some polemics. However it is generally agreed that these must have originated from the members of A-complement. One earliest explanation assumed that occasional nondisjunction simply gave rise to a 8-chromosome gamete and so on, but this can be rejected for the fact that plants with B-chromosomes do not show any trisomic or tetrasomic behaviour. An alternative explanation, first offered by GOTOH (1924), and later supported by STOLZE (1925), EMME (1927), DARLINGTON (1933) and others, is based on the assumption that transverse segmentation through the centromere region gave rise to telocentrics that could be perpetuated after some alterations. On the other hand, LAMM (1936) supported NAVASHIN's (1934) view that some complex fragmentation occurred by the breakage of chromatin bridges during first meiotic division followed by nondisjunction in second to give rise to 8-chromosome gametes. Perhaps one still more plausible suggestion is that of STUTZ (1957), originally hinted by POPOFF in 1939, according to which interspecific hybridization might have been involved. To be precise, STUTZ suggested that crossingover between a terminal segment of a *cereale* chromosome and an interstitial region of a *montanum* chromosome would result in a subterminal and smaller chromosome. That such a crossover is not an impossible event, is in agreement with the finding that there are some duplications present in the karyotypes of these species. Accordingly, one may expect to find the Turkish populations with higher frequency of B-chromosomes since both species grow together in this region.

MÜNTZING (1950) however stated that in rye, the origin of B-chromosomes remains completely obscure. One argument against the hypothesis of interspecific hybridization is that in Swedish strains standard fragment seems to have been arising continuously while there is no chance of such natural crossing in Sweden. Besides, MÜNTZING and LIMA-DE-FARIA's researches have shown that although a complete identity between standard fragment and any of the A-chromosomes is lacking, the fundamental pattern of their organization is alike and that it seems improbable to have involved another species in the origin of this fragment.

However, aside from the problem of their origin, there also remains the question of evolutionary significance: Do these accessory chromosomes play some role in the evolution and otherwise what genetic mechanism insures their perpetuation in a given entity? Admittedly as it stands today, these questions are largely unanswered. ÖSTERGREN (1947) believed that B-chromosomes must possess some special cycle of evolution based on what he designated as "genetic accumulation mechanisms". Their nondisjunctional mode of increase and some recent work by BOSEMARK (1957) indicates that they have a selective value and therefore some importance in evolution.

D. HAPLOIDY AND POLYPLOIDY

1. Haploids.

An important source of natural haploids is apomoxis (in broad sense) such as through polyembryony, parthenogenesis, or very rarely by the development of sperm nucleus entering the embryosac. AASE (1946) compiled a huge number of such cases reported in cereal crop species and he concluded that polyembryony has been a fairly good source of haploids as well as triploids. MÜNTZING (1937a; 1938) and SENGBUSCH (1940) examined a large number of heteroploid twins in rye among which a very small frequency of haploids was found. SENGBUSCH (1940), for instance, got only one case among 654 twins of both identical and fraternal types. KOSTOFF (1939a) had failed to find any among 20393 seedlings of Vjatka rye and about 40,000 offsprings of *cereale* × *montanum* crosses. This led him to believe that in a crossfertilized species, haploids would be soon eliminated due to the mutational 'load' of recessive lethals (or sublethals) characteristically present in their natural populations. But recently ZIMMERMANN (1951) succeeded in getting 7 haploids among only 348 twins he had analysed. Obviously it appears that the occurrence of haploidy and so also the 'twinning' vary from one strain to another, perhaps even from one genotype to another.

There are several methods known by which haploidy can be artificially induced. MÜNTZING (1937b) and NORDENSKIÖLD (1939) have reported successful induction in rye. By subjecting spikes to -3°C for 30 minutes after artificial pollinations and repeating this treatment every six hours, MÜNTZING (1937b) could obtain a haploid presumably by inducing parthenogenesis, that did not survive until maturity. NORDENSKIÖLD (1939) gave high temperature shock and in the haploid she observed meiotic irregularities as expected but she also found that about 3% of the PMC's had one rod bivalent, the average chiasma frequency per cell being 0.03. These data did not seem to be of any great interest.

LEVAN (1942) carried out a detailed cytological study of three of the natural haploids selected from among the twins by MÜNTZING. A typical pachytene was observed with pairing often initiating at the heterochromatic end knobs and at diplotene or diakinesis. LEVAN recorded bivalents and occasionally also a trivalent. The average chiasma frequency per cell varied (range 0.08–0.83) among these three plants. This 'intrahaploid' pairing (DARLINGTON, 1937) is not necessarily same as the nonhomologous pairing first described by McCLINTOCK (1933). She had pointed out that two chromosomes homologous for a greater part could pair even in nonhomologous regions under the tension of pairing in adjacent segments. In order to account for as much pairing as two bivalents plus a trivalent observed by LEVAN in a few cells, a good deal of homology, or affinity due to some other reason, will have to be assumed and as LIMA-DE-FARIA (1952b). points out, it is rather difficult to see how such a convergent type of chromosome evolution may have taken place in rye. Therefore, it seems very desirable to obtain more information about the cytology of haploids, trisomics and various aneuploids [1]. NAKAJIMA (1952) suggested that haploidy may be studied in diploid *Triticum* × *Secale* hybrids (2n = 21 or 28).

2. *Triploids.*

By selection among a large population of heteroploid twins, MÜNTZING (1938) could isolate two triploids. No cytological work seems to have been reported by him. KOSTOFF (1939) obtained a triploid which he believed to have arisen from endosperm cell. His data showed that

---

[1]) It will be noted that in case of rye, there are only few things to which this clause does not apply. For instance, information on interspecific hybridization, population genetics and linkage maps is also badly needed.

often 2–4 trivalents formed and both pollen and seed fertility were very poor. LAMM (1944) found a relatively higher degree of pairing in his triploid plant (mean number of trivalents and univalents per cell were 3.75 ± 0.36 and 3.25 ± 0.37 respectively) and a minimum of 25% chromosome elimination resulting in pollen grains with 9–10 chromosomes (average), larger in size and completely sterile. On pollinating with pollen from a normal diploid, he obtained a few seeds, all diploids. Besides these data there is no other report of cytological nature in literature known to the present writer. BRESLAVETZ (1940) succeeded in getting one triploid plant of spring rye during the course of his colchicine investigations and showed cell size in it to be intermediate between that of diploid and a tetraploid. Several attempts to obtain triploids by crossing 2n and 4n individuals have met with total failure (embryological studies mentioned in a later section).

3. Trisomics.

The papers by KOSTOFF (1937) and KOSTOFF *et al* (1935) reported only the occurrence of some trisomics in the progeny of *cereale* × *montanum* hybrids. TAKAGI (1935) has studied the cytology of a trisomic plant that originated from an openpollinated spike of the material and that GOTOH (1932) seemed to consider as having an accessory chromosome. However, from TAKAGI's drawings it appears that this extra chromosome is the regular SAT-chromosome and that the plant is indeed a trisomic case. At diakinesis, PMC's with 6 II and I III were nearly as frequent as those with 7II and one I whereas at first metaphase a few cells had also 6II + 3I thus giving slightly lower figure for average chiasma frequency too. On account of there being no visible morphological differences from diploids, TAKAGI was led to erroneous conclusion that the SAT-chromosome was genetically inactive. (Studies by RILEY and CHAPMAN (1957) have obtained valuable data on this issue and will be referred to again in Section IF). MÜNTZING and PRAKKEN (1941) carried out a cytological study of two trisomic individuals, both these also having the SAT-chromosome in triplicate, and besides a lower frequency of trivalent formation as compared to TAKAGI's data, they observed quite often only one satellite instead of three perhaps because the nucleolar organization involved only one or two of them except in a case where the freelying univalent seemed to form its own small nucleolus. It may be added here in passing that some workers disagree with each other about a direct correlation between the number of secondary constrictions and that of nucleoli formed (see GATES, 1942, for instance).

LIMA-DE-FARIA (1952b) suggested a possible use of trisomic plant studies in connection with the problem of genetic differentiation, or homology, that may exist between the chromosomes of rye comple- ment. Accordingly, there will be expected fewer than seven distinct trisomic types if the genetic differentiation was any markedly in- complete. The importance of this sort of information can not be overemphasized.

4. Tetraploids.

a) Incidence in nature. In rye, a good number of naturally oc- curring autotetraploids could be isolated and subsequently propagated from among the twins, triplets or quadruplets (MÜNTZING, 1938; SENGBUSCH, 1940). Many other euploid variants in nature, unless shown to be arising from mitotic accidents in various vegetative tissues in which case the polyploidy may cover only a few sex cells (LEVAN, 1942) or a larger sector of tissues (MÜNTZING and PRAKKEN, 1941) giving chimaeras, remain of an obscure origin. LAMM (1936) and MÜNTZING (1936) also observed such polyploid sectors involving an entire anther or only parts of its loculi. A famous tetraploid strain called Rosen rye was derived from a diploid-tetraploid chimaera discovered in Swedish variety, Östgota Gråråg (MÜNTZING, 1938). A case of spontaneous chromosome doubling during the seedling stage was recorded by O'MARA (1943). However, since colchicine induction is much more convenient source, it appears natural that attempts to search for natural polyploids may have been only few.

b) Induction experiments. The use of colchicine has been made by rye workers with variable degree of success, and this might be accounted for by such factors as the method of treatment, dosage of the chemical and possibly also the material used. Table 3 below gives a summary of results of these experiments. Thus it appears that placing germinating seeds in aqueous solutions (0.1 to 0.2%) gave good results. However, the present writer failed to obtain any healthy seedlings from treatments with these relatively high concentrations. The root- tips had swollen and on cytological examination showed polyploid cells but the plants showed no further growth after about a week.

The concentrations used and the duration of treatment seem to be very critical. A promising method of treating grass seedlings or clonal divisions was suggested by STEBBINS (1949) and might be tried in rye too. Besides colchicine, a few other agents have been tried with some

TABLE 3. Colchicine experiments for inducing polyploidy in rye.

Material	Method of treatment and dosage	Remarks	Reference
Spring rye	Seeds germinated in pulp made of Colchicum plants	Unsuccessful	KOSTOFF (1939)
Winter rye	Seeds germinated in 0.05–0.025% solutions	,,	MÜNTZING and RUNQVIST (1939)
Spring rye	Germinating seeds placed in solutions	Fairly effective	BRESLAVETZ (1939)
Winter rye	Germinating seeds immersed after removing young coleoptile. 0.02 to 0.1% for 24 hrs.	Highly successful	KONDO (1941)
,,	Ears immersed in solution	,,	LI (cited after CHIN, 1943)
,,	Seeds germinated in solutions	Fairly successful	SENGBUSCH (1940)
,,	Seeds germinated and placed in solutions, 0.2% for 2 hrs. or 0.1% for 3 hrs.	Highly successful ,,	BREMER-REINDERS and BREMER (1952)
Both spring and winter rye	(i) Seeds treated soon after pre-soaking in water; 0.1%, 2 days.	Less effective	BRAGDO (1955)
,,	(ii) seedlings dipped in 0.2% solution for 20 mins.	Highly successful	,,

success. Those include the heat shock (DORSEY, 1936), Roentgen rays (BRESLAVETZ, 1939; BRESLAVETZ *et al*, 1935) and brome-acenaphthene and brome-naphthaline (SCHMUCK and KOSTOFF, 1939). BRAVO (1956) used lindane on germinating seeds at 0.5, 1.0 and 1.5% concentrations and obtained some sectors with restitution nuclei.

   c) Meiotic studies. Autopolyploids are characterized and indeed identified by the presence of multivalents formed at first metaphase of meiosis. As often is the case, in autotretraploids of rye also the frequency of quadrivalents is found to vary within as well as between plants. MÜNTZING and PRAKKEN (1941) analysed 24 cells in the tetraploid spikes of a 2n/4n chimaera and of them 4 had 2 IV plus one III, 7 had 2–3 IV and the average quadrivalent frequency per cell was 2.33 (range 0–6). MÜNTZING (1951a) and MORRISON 1956) obtained the corresponding figures as 3.81 and 4.05 respectively and this variation might be explained on the basis of differences in the material and conditions of fixation together with the sampling errors. CHIN (1943) however obtained an exceptionally low figure of 0.71 IV per cell which could hardly be accounted for by his data on chiasma frequencies and terminalization coefficient that were lower in case of tetraploids than the diploids. Likewise the averages for trivalent and univalent frequency differed in the materials studied by these workers (e.g. MÜNTZING, 1951a, 0.14 III and 0.28 I per cell; CHIN, 1943, 0.34 III and 1.10 I per cell). Moreover, while O'MARA (1943) had found occasional interlocked quadrivalents, others observed only zigzag or nonzigzag, simple configurations (MÜNTZING and PRAKKEN, 1941; CHIN, 1943; PLARRE 1953, 1954).

The relative counts of different types of segregation could only be studied in the form of transmission of aneuploidy and not much seems to have been done so far in rye, and for that matter, in most other autopolyploids. However, from the high pollen fertility of rye tetraploids, it would appear that segregation is perhaps often regular. The behaviour of univalents is typically thus: they divide at first anaphase, lag behind during the second anaphase and thus often make appearance as micronuclei in tetrads or pollen grains (CHIN, 1943; MÜNTZING, 1951; BREMER and BREMER-REINDERS, 1954; PLARRE, 1954; MORRISON, 1956). O'MARA (1943) noted a number of bridges at anaphase I some of which he thought to be explicable on the basis of structural heterozygosity. He also reported some PMC's singly or in groups to have hypoploid chromosome numbers presumably as a result of chromosome elimination at some preceding stage. MÜNTZING (1951b), on the other hand, observed small chromatin (?) dots in the cytoplasm of many cells at first anaphase or telophase. In general, meiotic irregularities in tetraploids of rye are similar to those found in many others.

d) Pollen and seed fertility. KONDO (1941) recorded on an average 60–70% pollen fertility in his tetraploid material while as high as

95% (PLARRE, 1954; MORRISON, 1956) and 96.9% (CHIN, 1943) are also on record in literature. In comparison with diploids, an overall average figure of 15–25% reduction in pollen fertility may serve as good approximation. Ovular fertility is relatively much more variable and may be lowered in the range of 20 to 70% of the original values. This might at first seem to hold contrary to a generally known fact that egg cells are less affected by many chromosomal irregularities, but here the causes of sterility are of both haplontic and diplontic nature. HÅKANSSON and ELLERSTRÖM (1950) however argued that since higher seed sterility in tetraploids was due to either increase in failure of fertilization, or an increase in the frequency of cases showing slow, incomplete zygote development, the haplontic causes had only secondary importance. MÜNTZING (1946b, 1949) observed occasionally small embryosacs, more commonly in tetraploids, with underdeveloped antipodals that apparently failed to complete development. Furthermore, it was shown that development of embryo as well as endosperm in general was slower than in diploids (HÅKANSSON and ELLERSTRÖM, 1950) which could be primarily due to lower rates of nuclear division.

SENGBUSCH (1941) brought out another important feature of seed sterility in tetraploid rye. From his study of colchicine – induced tetraploids for three successive years, he demonstrated the fact that there results higher seed set if tetraploid material was grown in isolation from diploids which later investigations showed to be due to the factor of triploid embryo failure (MÜNTZING, 1943; BLEIER, 1950; HÅKANSSON and ELLERSTRÖM, 1950; LÖWENSTEIN, 1951; PLARRE, 1954; ELLERSTRÖM and HÅGBERG, 1954; KOO, 1958). CHIN (1943) studied the pollen tube growth in reciprocal crosses between diploids and tetraploids and found the diploid pollen as giving rise to abortive tubes in diploid styles. He pointed out further that in mixed pollinations with haploid and diploid pollen, the former was more effective selectively which in this case, was apparently not related to heteromorphy. HÅKANSSON and ELLERSTRÖM (1950), on the contrary, observed that fertilization readily succeeded in both combinations, i.e. 4n ♀ × 2n ♂ and its reciprocal, and that the initial zygote development was apparently normal. On fourth and sixth day after fertilization, the endosperm showed differences from the controls, that is 2n × 2n and 4n × 4n pollinations, and also

they found a marked difference between the two reciprocal combinations (4n × 2n and 2n × 4n). The former of these appeared to be
normal so far while in the case of latter, mitotic irregularities were
seen in endosperm tissue; however, in both endosperm eventually
disintegrates and embryo dies. According to LÖWENSTEIN (1951),
some kind of physiological unbalance among the antipodal, maternal,
embryo and endosperm tissue constitution was causing the total
failure of triploid zygotes. Thus it is significant to note that for a
hybrid to be successful during these stages not only the genetic constitution of its parents but their ability to produce an endosperm
capable of providing adequate nourishment to the embryo alongwith
harmony among the tissues of mother individual, embryo and endosperm is very critical (STEBBINS, 1958).

There have been made attempts to improve seed setting of tetraploid rye through selection, and some attention given also to the
presence of aneuploids (2n = 26, 27, 29, 30 and 31 have been found
not infrequently) in tetraploid populations. Of these, cases of 2n = 27,
29 are relatively much more common. MÜNTZING (1943b) showed that
aneuploids set mostly shrivelled seed so that through seed selection
on a large scale, they could be eliminated, or at least thinned down to
a minimum. On an average, he (1951) found 22.7% plants of original
population to be aneuploids, higher chromosome numbers being in
a majority. The frequency of aneuploids varies greatly among different populations (HÅGBERG, 1953; BREMER and BREMER-REINDERS,
1954) and the following few data (Table 4) from BREMER and BREMER-

TABLE 4. Data of BREMER and BREMER-REINDERS (1954): (See text)

Year	% Regular cells at anaphase I (without laggards)	% of aneuploids among progeny of selected seeds	% seed set of population
First	66.9	24.50	60% or less
Third	75.0	12.16	
Sixth	87.0	7.40	75% or more

REINDERS (1954) shows the amount of improvement these workers
could obtain after six generations of selection. Their cytological data
on the relative frequencies of irregular anaphase I, metaphase II and
tetrads also indicate a progressive increase in regularity of meiotic

behaviour. PLARRE (1954) indeed selected on the basis of meiotic behaviour and after a few generations of selection he obtained about 5–8% increase in fertility and therefore higher yields.

Thus it seems obvious that meiotic behaviour is correlated with seed fertility of tetraploids. However, environment might have an important role to play as can be inferred from the fact that tetraploid rye grown at Davis, California, does very well (SUNESON, unpublished) and recently HÅGBERG and his collaborators have taken up cytological investigations in this material. HILPERT (1957) has reported his selection experiments in tetraploid summer strains. He arrived at conclusion that while one year's selection gave no significant effect, further work would improve meiotic regularity and seed set as well as seed quality. It may be noted here that MORRISON (1956) believes any such improvement to be due to genetic causes or physiological changes, rather than chromosome behaviour. However, MÜNTZING (1951b, 1956) is hopeful of large scale utilization of tetraploid rye in near future and he reported that "in various combinations between tetraploid varieties of rye strong degrees of heterosis have been observed, leading to increases in kernel yield ranging from 15–20 percent".

e) *General effects of tetraploidy.* Autotetraploid rye possesses all general characteristics observed among other species. Its 'gigas' nature has been shown by increase in size of epidermal and stomatal cells (BRESLAVETZ, 1939, 1940; KONDO, 1941; CHIN, 1943), thicker roots (PETERS, 1954), thicker culms (NAKAJIMA, 1954d), longer and broader leaves (PLARRE, 1953, 1954) and larger pollen grains (BRAGDO, 1955, and others cited above) as compared to the diploids. As STEBBINS (1950, p. 303) pointed out, all other gigas characteristics might be related to one primary difference, that is of cell size, and likewise the differences in cell content of various substances such as protein, chlorophyll and water might be only secondary effects. LEVAN (1947) found in tetraploids a lower pigment content per unit of green weight and similarly papers by NOGGLE (1947) and HINTZER and MIRANDA (1954) report differences with respect to total nitrogen content, reducing sugars, carotene, riboflavine and ascorbic acid. As illustrations of growth retardation effects may be mentioned reports of reduction in stem length (PLARRE, 1954), tillering capacity (MÜNTZING, 1951a) and spikelet number (PLARRE, 1954).

One most important feature of tetraploid rye is the grain weight (or thousand grain weight) which is about 50% higher than in diploid rye (MÜNTZING, 1951a; SCHILDT and ÅKERBERG, 1951; TJIO and SANCHEZ-MONGE, 1954; PLARRE, 1954). Among others on record in literature are better sprouting ability (MÜNTZING, 1951a), reduced shattering before harvest perhaps due to larger glume size (PLARRE, 1954), superior baking ability (MÜNTZING, 1951a; HINTZER and MIRANDA, 1954), higher sensitivity to vernalization and photoperiodic treatment (LAUBE, 1956) but greater resistance to the effects of Roentgen rays and temperature shocks (BRESLAVETZ *et al*, 1935; SMITH, 1943). LUNDQVIST (1947, 1953, 1956), LÖWENSTEIN (1951) and PLARRE (1954) studied the self-incompatibility status of tetraploids and their findings seem to be in agreement. In Stålråg, LUNDQVIST found that tetraploids were unaffected as regards self-sterility but showed some improvement in self-compatibility.

E. INTERSPECIFIC HYBRIDIZATION

Of all the cytogenetic features that one finds perhaps most interesting in the study and description of a given genus, interspecific hybridization occupies a unique place and this seems very natural in view of its bearing on our understanding of genetics and evolution. However, in *Secale* very little work has been done on interspecific hybrids except for that just started within past 8–10 years. Nevertheless, it will be apparent from below that such investigations have proven very rewarding. For the sake of convenience in following review, it may be pointed out here that all known species in this genus have been classified by ROSHEVITZ (1948) into three sections, namely *Cerealia* (includes cultivated or weedy annuals), *Sylvestria* (wild, annual- *S. sylvestre* being the only one) and *Kuprijanovii* (all perennials). Now, since early workers seem to have been primarily interested in the transfer of such characters as perenniality and hardiness from wild to cultivated species, hybrids between members of same section apparently offered no interest to them. KOSTOFF (1931, 1932) however reported his study of three combinations, *cereale* × *ancestrale*, *cereale* × *vavilovii** and *ancestrale* × *vavilovii**, in all of them F_1 showing regular meiosis with seven bivalents forming at metaphase I except for occasional cell having two univalents. He found their fertility as high as in parents (about 90%) and also indication of hybrid vigour. NAKAJIMA (1956) too reports *cereale* × *vavilovi** to be having regular meiotic behaviour and fertility. (* these crosses involving some material believed to be *vavilovii* are interpreted below in light of writer's own results). Two more intrasection species hybrids are on record: those are between members of *Kuprijanovii*. SCHIE-MANN and KRÜGER (1952) in *montanum* × *africanum* and its recipro-cal, RILEY (1956) in *montanum* × *dalmaticum* and STEBBINS and JAIN (unpub.) in *africanum* × *vavilovii* observed F_1 having regular seven bivalents formed during meiosis with only occasional cases of univalents being present. However, in the last hybrid mentioned there were observed a relatively high occurrence of irregular anaphase cells and of microspores having micronuclei.

Among the hybrids between annual and perennial species, *cereale* × *montanum* cross has been studied by many workers. TSCHERMAK (1906 and later) initiated genetic studies in rye with this hybrid which he reported to be moderately fertile and as having most of *montanum* characters. LONGLEY and SANDO (1930) and also ANTONOFF (1936) and NAKAJIMA (1954) reported in it meiosis to be quite regular with all seven bivalents formed normally. The results of KOSTOFF (1937) differed slightly in that he found in F_1 5–7 bivalents and reduction of fertility. Occasionally these workers found cells having non-synchronous anaphase separation, multivalent formation and chromo-somes lagging at anaphase I. KOSTOFF (1937) further studied the backcross to *cereale* parent and this he found to have greater vigour and fertility. But contrary to the remarks by him and others, SMITH (1942) reported only about 26–27% pollinations being successful. Among other primarily genetic studies on *cereale* × *montanum* hy-brids may be mentioned those of REZNUICK (1931), OSSENT (1930) and DUKA (1935, 1936).

However, it was left for SCHIEMANN and NURNBERG-KRÜGER (1952) to record a discovery of unusual interest in their study of *cereale* × *montanum* and *cereale* × *africanum* hybrids. At metaphase I, the maximum association was found to be a translocation configu-ration, chain-of-six, indicating that since *montanum* × *africanum* gave only bivalents, the *cereale* chromosome complement must have been different from both *montanum* and *africanum* by the presence of two reciprocal translocations between them. At anaphase about

12–15% of PMC's showed various irregularities and the hybrids were poor in fertility. These observations soon stimulated further investigations (PRICE, 1955a, b; RILEY, 1956; STUTZ, 1957). That *cereale-montanum* hybrids provide very useful material for a study of the nature and causes of hybrid sterility was pointed out by PRICE (1955b) who was studying crosses between *S. cereale* (Merced variety) and two different strains of *S. montanum*, coded as 'Copenhagen' and 'Iran' according to the source of their seed-collection, and using normal as well as irradiated pollen. His cytological observations confirmed the regular occurrence of a chain-of-six configuration and other above-mentioned characteristics of this hybrid, and further he noted that chromosome alterations present in r-hybrids (i.e. using irradiated pollen) were of same kind as in the control hybrids (i.e. using normal pollen as usual) except for some new induced translocations, small inversions or occasional fragmentation. In r-hybrids therefore some cells showed a chain-of-eight as the maximum association. However, PRICE (1955b) could establish in both instances a lack of significant correlation between the frequency of various meiotic irregularities and pollen fertility. In addition, some evidence for the prevalence of genic causes of sterility observed in this hybrid was obtained from a statistical analysis of within and between family mean differences. Accordingly, a complementary model similar to one putforth by DOBZHANSKY (1951) was suggested by PRICE who also held the opinion that sterility barrier between these species was in an incipient stage.

Another form of at least partial reproductive barrier between these species with different chromosome arrangement types was noted by RILEY (1956) who found hybrid seed of crosses between *cereale* and *montanum* (or *dalmaticum*) germinable only when *cereale* was the female parent. While meiosis in *montanum* × *dalmaticum* hybrid was regular with its seven bivalents formed during first metaphase, in their hybrids with *cereale*, cells with trivalents, quadrivalents, quinque- and sexivalents occurred with only slight differences in relative frequencies. RILEY (1956) observed two cases, one with a chain-of-eight and another with chain-of-five plus a chain-of-three, indicating a third translocation difference to be also present and to explain the rarity of such associations he assumed that either interchange segments of this translocation must be small, or occurred in a region where chiasma frequency was low. From his study of F_2, RILEY seemed to obtain the segregation of translocation patterns in original parental combination so that he was led to infer that certain factors present in the median regions of three chromosome pairs that are involved in translocation configuration, might probably have an adaptive value thus tending to maintain species differentiation. Referring to the influence of breeding systems on the role of translocations in evolution (WRIGHT, 1940), it was pointed out that in this case fluctuations in population size might have had significant effects. However, STUTZ (1957) studying *cereale × montanum* cross obtained evidence for a cross-over to be taking place in the differential segment as well which discredits RILEY's assumption of any morphological features associated with species identity being preserved through translocations. STUTZ also carried out a detailed analysis of the configuration-of-six chromosomes (no case of higher multivalents was noted among his or present writer's material). Observations on most frequent diakinetic configurations allowed an identification of each of the chromosomes involved and at least by inference the relative size and the position of interchange segments. His results further indicated the presence of a deficiency in median region and a terminal duplication in one of these chromosomes. It is interesting to note that the expected maximum configuration, ring-of-six, occurred only occasionally and seemed to have dissociated at a particular pair of chromosome ends, as could be shown by the fact that often the knobbed chromosome of cereale arrangement was observed at the end of resulting chain. The original paper should be consulted for a lucid discussion of these findings. In F_2 STUTZ observed the modal association to be chain-of-four that he interprets to be a product of adjacent disjunction in the translocation configuration, a situation made possible by the presence of duplications. Also he recorded in a number of F_2 segregants presence of an extra chromosome belonging to the translocation group. This suggests a possible mode of origin of certain types of B-chromosomes.

Recently a number of other interspecific hybrids have been cytologically studied (STEBBINS and JAIN, unpub.) and the results are summarily given below in Table 5. (See also Fig. 9–12).

It should be pointed out that in both hybrids involving *sylvestre* as one of the parents, the frequency of chains-of-six was found to be less than in other three translocation heterozygotes listed below in Table 5. Instead, there occurred quadrivalents much more frequently. On the other hand, in the case of Transcaucasian × *vavilovii* hybrid one plant gave three metaphase I cells with ring-of-six, the maximum

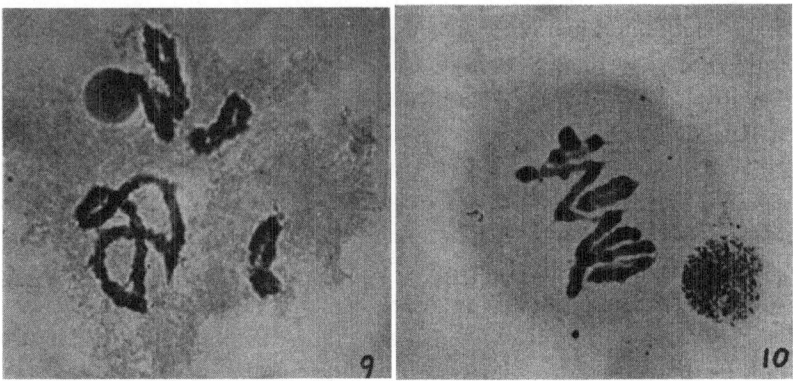

Figs. 9–10. Typical cells of translocation heterozygotes to show a ring-of-six at diakinesis and a chain-of-six at M I. See text.

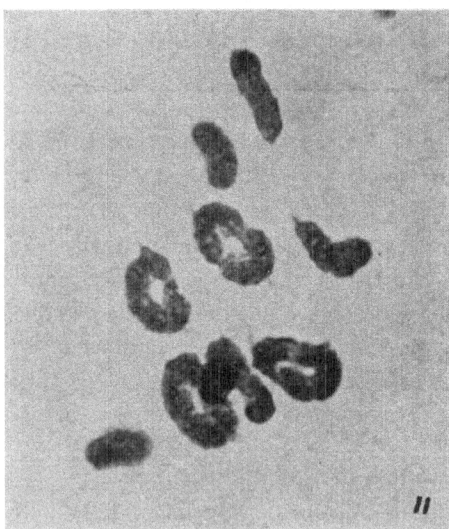

Fig. 11. A metaphase I plate in *vavilovii* × *sylvestre* hybrid to show the occurrence of univalents. (See Table 5).

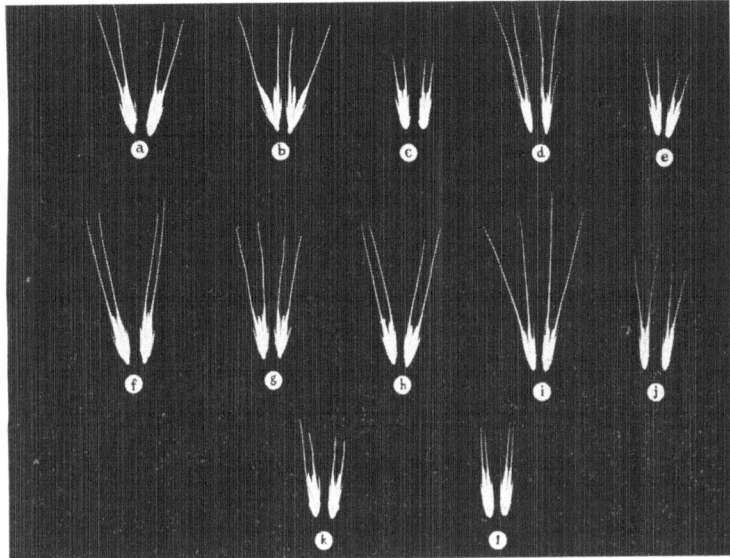

Fig. 12. Spikelets of species and species hybrids. a-Transcaucasian rye; b-cereale; c-vavilovii; d-sylvestre; e-africanum. f, g-Trans. × cereale, and reciprocal; h-cer. × vav.; i-vav. × sylv.; j-afr. × sylv.; k-Trans. × vav.; l-Trans. × afr. Note the characteristic glume beak of *sylvestre* appearing in both hybrids involving it.

TABLE 5. Cytology of some interspecific hybrids studied by STEBBINS and JAIN (unpub.)

Cross ♀ ♂	Metaphase I (mean per cell)			Pollen fert. %
	I (Uni.)	II (Biv.)	VI (Sexiv.)	
cer. × Trans.*	0.26	6.87	—	87,49
Trans.* × cer.	0.20	6.90	—	89.26
afr. × vav.	0.48	6.76	—	(no data taken)
afr. × sylv.	1.73	4.60	0.07	15.35
vav. × sylv.	2.25	3.77	0.10	9.74
cer. × vav.	0.40	4.46	0.45	16.86
Trans* × afr.	0.54	4.67	0.39	15.04
Trans* × vav.	0.39	4.43	0.54	11.38

(* At this point it is necessary to comment on *vavilovii* material used in these crosses. Trans. refers to a rye strain received from the Department of Armenian Flora, S. Transcaucasia, and labelled as vavilovii. However, the material referred to as *vavilovii* in above Table was collected by Prof. Dr. H. KUCKUCK from Hamadan, Iran, and has been identified so with the original description of GROSSHEIM (1924). Therefore it appears that KOSTOFF (1931) and NAKAJIMA (1956) might have used some strain similar to this Transcaucasian rye as *vavilovii*).

expected association on basis of two translocations. Thus it might indicate the presence of some additional 'cryptic' structural differences in respect with homology between these species although these translocations form a major difference in all five hybrids. Figure 13

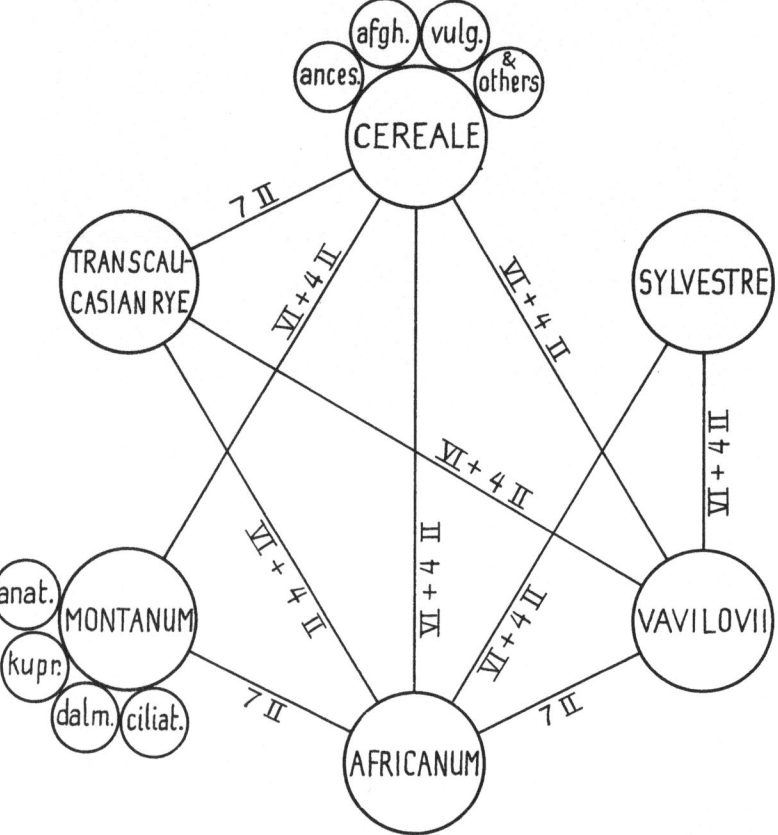

Fig. 13. Chart showing pairing relationships known among the interspecific hybrids. Note that on this basis, two distinct chromosome arrangement types are represented by *cereale-sylvestre* and *montanum-africanum-vavilovii* respectively. *ancestrale, afghanicum, vulgare*, etc. are tentatively considered as varieties of *cereale*, and similarly, *anatolicum, Kuprijanovii, dalmaticum* and *ciliatoglume* of *montanum*.

shows diagrammatically the pairing situation in all known interspecific hybrids of genus *Secale* and further emphasizes how *cereale-sylvestre*-Transcaucasian rye on one hand and *montanum-africanum-*

vavilovii on the other form two distinct groups in this respect. These findings are briefly discussed elsewhere for their bearing on the problem of the origin of cultivated rye and systematics of this genus. (Sections III & IV). Further work should be taken up with most of these and other interspecific hybrids, both from cytological and genetical viewpoints. At present, for example, almost nothing is known about the exact nature of translocation differences between other species than *cereale* and *montanum* as to whether same segments were involved in each instance; or about the behaviour of F_2 generation with respect to chromosomal or genetic segregation.

F. INTERGENERIC HYBRIDIZATION

Intergeneric hybridization is perhaps most strikingly represented in Tribe *Hordeae* (*GRAMINEAE*) which is comprised of following ten genera: *Aegilops, Agropyron, Elymus, Haynaldia, Heteranthelicum, Hordeum, Hystrix, Secale, Sitanion* and *Triticum*. STEBBINS and his associates have extensively studied both artificial and natural hybrids between members of several of them (STEBBINS, 1950, for earlier references; STEBBINS and SNYDER, 1956; and STEBBINS, 1956). Briefly, these researches have presented evidence to suggest a radical change in the systematics of this Tribe such as often categorized under 'lumping'. In below the work on hybridization involving rye will be briefly reviewed.

1. With Triticum.

An impressive amount of literature exists on the research work in wheat-rye hybrids. However, since O'MARA (1953) has recently reviewed all of its major aspects it will be necessary to mention here only a few more important ones and some results reported in recent years.

It may be recalled that breeders' main interest in wheat-rye hybrids aims at the exploitation of some useful rye characters such as winter hardiness, disease and insect pest resistance or low soil fertility requirements so that all endeavour has been directed to either producing suitable amphiploids, or transferring specific character through chromosome addition or substitution. Some studies on genom homologies were stimulated by MEISTER's (1925) postulate of hexaploid wheats having originated from *Triticum dicoccum* × *Secale cereale* hybrids. These three lines of investigations are briefly mentioned below.

The cytological reports on a variety of *Triticum* × *Secale* hybrids are too numerous to be included in this list here but it is significant to note that the number of bivalent associations at first metaphase has been found to vary from none (LONGLEY and SANDO, 1930), 1 to 2 (ZALENSKY and DOROSHENKO, 1925; BLEIER, 1930), three (KIHARA, 1924; THOMPSON, 1926; AASE, 1930), to as many as four (BLEIER, 1940; NAKAJIMA, 1952a) and even six (KATTERMANN, 1938b). In general, more than three bivalents were observed when *T. sphaero-coccum* was used instead of *T. vulgare (aestivum)*. However, except for KAGAWA and CHIZAKI (1934) who believed that two of the five bivalents found in *T. durum* × *S. cereale* were heterogenetic associ-ations (the terms auto-and allo-syndesis have been carefully inter-preted by STEBBINS, 1950, since until now these were frequently misused), others have held the opinion of all association being homo-genetic and within wheat complement, again with single exception reported by NAKAJIMA (1952a) who explains 11 bivalents as including 7 among A and B genoms, one within D genome and 3 of rye genome. NAKAJIMA has extensively published his results in almost all hybrid combinations between *Secale cereale, montanum, africanum* and *vavilovii* on one hand and several representatives of Emmer and *vulgare* wheats (NAKAJIMA, 1942, 1948, 1950a, b, 1952b, 1953a–c, and others cited in bibliography). He found the percentage of successful pollinations was notably high in case of *T. vulgare* × *S. cereale*, *T. compactum* × *S. cereale*, *T. sphaerococcum* × *S. africanum* and *T. sphaerococcum* × *S. vavilovii*, and in most cases the hybrid closely resembled the wheat parent. Metaphase I pairing ranged from 0 to four bivalents, with only a few exceptions, and fertility from 0 to about 20 per cent.

VILLAX and MOTA (1953) reported an unusual observation as they found in their wheat × rye hybrid material a spike giving 48-chromo-some plants that on treating with colchicine, resembled at maturity the wheat parent and they postulated rye chromosomes to have been lost at some stage during treatment. LEISER (1954) analyzed 59 differ-ent lines that comprised of amphiploids (2n = 56) as well as many hypoploid derivatives (2n = 48 to 54). A majority of them looked intermediate between their parental phenotypes but for three dominant rye characters namely, the pubescence of peduncle (also known as hairy-neck), lodging resistance and resistance to rust and mildew. Further he established a relationship between the fertility and meiotic regularity in amphiploids and by crossing primary (i.e. 28-chromosome) hybrids to amphiploids (*Triticale*) he could obtain 42-chromosome plants that seemed to be useful material for genetic transfer studies. SANCHEZ-MONGE (1956) attempted about 300 cross combinations between different emmer wheats and *cereale* rye that resulted after colchicine treatment in nine 48-chromosome plants and from their progeny he (1957) has been able to derive polyhaploid types. MÜNTZING (1955), on the other hand, obtained 70-chromosome types by crossing *Triticale*, 2n = 56, with diploid rye parent and again doubling the chromosome number so that these strains represent (42 + 28) combination of wheat and tetraploid rye. However, in all these cases the sanguine hope of immediate economic utilization has met the difficulty of poor yielding ability, again as in the case of autotetraploid rye the seed fertility being affected.

Several explanations have been forwarded for this sterility in wheat-rye amphiploids and disturbed chromosome pairing. They are briefly reviewed here.

(i) The chromosome number of Triticales is too large to allow normal and complete pairing. Studies of 42-chromosome amphiploids which also suffer from poor fertility, would hold against such a view (O'MARA, 1943; NAKAJIMA, 1952a).

(ii) There are present some specific antagonistic interactions between the rye chromosome carrying the hairy-neck factors and the chromosome IX of wheat (O'MARA, 1947). O'MARA found that while the addition of this rye pair into wheat complement gave badly affected plants, relatively normal individuals were obtained by adding some other pair. Accordingly, SEARS (1956) synthesized a nullisomic-IX amphiploid (2n = 54) which showed neither improved meiotic behaviour nor any better fertility than usual 56-chromosome amphiploids, so that O'MARA's (1947) view does not seem to hold valid.

(iii) ROSENSTIEL (1950) suggested that factors affecting the crossability between wheat and rye might also have an adverse effect on the meiotic behaviour of hybrids but SEARS (unpub.) has shown this to be rather unlikely because use of China Spring wheat which crosses readily gave no better fertile amphiploids.

(iv) Based on the assumption that infertility of amphiploids is directly relatable to the occurrence of univalents at metaphase I, MÜNTZING (1939) considered this asynaptic tendency to be due to the fact that in Triticale homozygous conditions are present while rye is an allogamous species. MÜNTZING and AKDIK (1948b) obtained evidence of the presence of recessive factors in rye populations that lowered pairing and fertility in derived inbreds. MÜNTZING (1951) further showed that amphiploids obtained from the use of rye inbreds were superior than those produced from open-pollinated rye parent. On the other hand, RILEY and CHAPMAN (1957) compared *Triticale* with *Triticum-Aegilops* amphiploids to show that least fertile ones were derived from among Triticales although *S. cereale* is outbreeder. Further evidence against MÜNTZING's hypothesis was obtained from studies on crosses between the amphiploids (O'MARA, 1953; RILEY and CHAPMAN, 1957). Furthermore, CHAPMAN and RILEY (1955) found that the 56-chromosome amphiploid had 28 bivalents in 40% of the pollen mother cells while the disomic addition derivatives (2n = 44) showed complete synapsis in only 9.7% cells and yet both equally infertile. LEBEDEFF's (1934) explanation based on the assumption of self-sterility factors of rye being responsible has also lacked experimental evidence so far.

KATTERMANN (1937, 1938b) obtained 42-chromosome hybrids from (wheat × rye) × *Triticale* cross and in them he observed perfect pairing in as many as 94% cells. Such a situation again seems unexplicable on basis of any of the above hypotheses. STEBBINS (1950, p. 226) discussed similar cases finally to conclude that "superimposed on the chromosomal sterility, the hybrid must have had a gene combination causing asynapsis or desynapsis, similar to those which arise as occasional mutations in good species".

Another line of practical approach has been the production of socalled "alien chromosome addition races or substitution races" in which the wheat-rye hybrid is backcrossed to wheat and subsequently through selfing and selection manipulations, these strains are derived. O'MARA (1940, 1946, 1951; full reference list may be found here) outlined these methods and also pointed out the possible use in locating genes of rye complement. He was able to show that the factor for hairy-neck which belongs to rye parent alone, was located on chromosome I (see also RILEY and CHAPMAN, 1958) while results of CHAPMAN and RILEY (1955) identified it with chromosome II which might be suggestive of both being involved. O'MARA (1940) using awnless wheat, and awned rye parents produced a disomic (2n = 44) addition line having striking differences from wheat in respect with awning, culm height, ear density and leaf colour. One plant with 2n = 47 (at M I showing 23 II + I) had both awnedness and hairy-neck so that both chromosomes carrying these unlinked factors might have been added. Still more interesting was the occurrence of derivatives having addition of isochromosomes corresponding to long or short arm separately (O'MARA, 1951). RILEY (1956) reported to have derived six of the possible seven disomic races and later four different linkage groups could be identified on basis of such characters as growth habit, plant height, ear shape and straw colour, resistance to yellow rust and mildew and grain appearance. It is hoped that work along these lines would prove very useful in studies of rye genetics.

JENSEN and KENT (1952) claimed to have successfully transferred leaf rust and mildew resistance of rye to their winter wheat material and finding no addition or substitution cytologically they assumed a reciprocal translation to have taken place, but however, even the transfer might be disputable according to ROSENSTIEL (1950) and O'MARA (1953) who feel that in many cases such 'transfers' could be merely due to contaminate crossing with other wheat varieties.

In connection with wheat-rye hybridization, two more features merit special mention here, namely the crossability as a heritable character and the crossing with rye used as mother parent. BLACK-HOUSE (1916) first pointed out that some combinations proved more successful in terms of the relative amount of successful pollinations and that this crossability was inherited as a recessive. GAINES and STEVENSON (1922) and BUCHINGER (1931) also observed that use of Rosen rye proved better than others, and data of TAYLOR and QUISEN-BERRY (1935) and LEIN (1943a) further confirmed this to be governed by one major recessive factor and at least one minor factor. That crossability is transferable among various wheat strains, was claimed by TAYLOR and QUISENBERRY (1935) whereas according to LEIN (1943a, b) the crossability expression depended upon the recovery of hybrids from wheat-rye crosses. Using different wheat species in his crosses, VASILIEV (1940) reported evidence of polymeric inheritance. The experimental work by SCHMUCK *et al* (1944) and HALL (1954), on the other hand, demonstrated that crossability could be increased simply by transplanting the young hybrid on to the rye endosperm which clearly suggests that some kind of relationship at the level of endosperm plays a critical role in determining the survival of hybrids.

These findings and the fact pointed out earlier that in most cases hybrids resembled the wheat parent, suggest that crosses with rye being mother parent might be of great interest, yet surprisingly enough, only few attempts seem to have been made. GAINES and STEVENSON (1922) reported one successful case and this plant resembled rye parent more than wheat notably with respect to ear shape, and awning. They found Rosen rye to be most compatible, succeeding in both directions of crossing. BUCHINGER (1931) asserted that first rye ♀ – wheat ♂ hybrid was obtained in 1925 by MEISTER and TIMINIAKOFF, and himself produced one from the cross Champagner rye ♀ – Bohara wheat ♂. This hybrid bloomed 24 days later than rye parent and showed hairy-neck, semiawnedness, sterile pollen but setting about 3 percent on pollination. KARPETZAN (1954) also recorded the success in both directions although more when wheat was used as seed parent. Further data will be needed before any inferences about the genetics of these cases can be drawn.

2. *With Aegilops.*

Hybridization between rye and *Aegilops triuncialis* as well as other *Aegilops* species used as seed parent is found to be readily successful (TSCHERMAK, 1913; LEIGHTY *et al* 1926; AASE, 1935; BERG, 1931; BUCHINGER, 1934; KAGAWA and CHIZAKI, 1934; and others). Hybrids that were studied by KARPECHENKO *et al* (1929) seemed to resemble *Aegilops* parent in such characteristics as black ear colour and fragile rachis and their seeds although shrivelled gave good germination. The only cytological data available are about the metaphase I pairing as follows: BERG (1931), 5–7 bivalents; no bivalent (OEHLER, cited after ISENBECK and ROSENSTIEL, 1950) and that 5 to 8 univalents appeared larger in size than the other chromosomes (KAGAWA and CHIZAKI, 1934). However, there does not seem to exist any genom homology between these two genera.

3. With Agropyron.

A number of papers reported successful hybridization between *Secale cereale* (mother parent) and *Agropyron intermedium* (pollen parent) (VERUSHKINE 1936; cited after SMITH 1942; LJUBIMOVA, 1937; SMITH, 1942; STEBBINS and PUN, 1953; GAUL, 1953), or *A. cristatum* (KRASNJUK, 1935, 1946; AASE, 1935; SMITH, 1942). Other species of *Agropyron* such as *repens, sibiricum, elongatum* and *trichophorum* have also been attempted. STEBBINS and PUN (1953) recorded I M association for the chromosomes of two parents separately (since rye chromosomes are larger in size such a distinction was possible) and they found that only in two out of 50 PMC's there was a rod bivalent formed between the chromosomes of *Secale* and *Agropyron*, whereas mean figures for total number of paired chromosomes per cell and the number involved in multivalent associations were 15.83 (range 15–21) and 3.24 (range 0–9) respectively. Data reported by GAUL (1953, 1954) also show that homogenetic association (intragenomic in view of complete non-homology between the genoms of *Secale* and *Agropyron*) was frequent within the *Agropyron intermedium* complement. He found on an average 6.1 bivalents, 1.3 trivalents and 0.02 quadrivalents per cell whereas using his following formula for calculating the potential number per cell of chromosomes paired (P),

$$P = \frac{X^2 + X - B}{(2X - B) \cdot Z},$$

where X = number of chiasmata counted in cells of a particular preparation, B = number of chromosomes involved in pairing and Z = total number of cells, he obtained P = 20 for his material, pseudo-associations being often a possible cause of bias in any such estimate. In conclusion, GAUL affirms that *Secale* genome occupies isolated position in *Triticineae*. However, according to STEBBINS and PUN (1953) these relationships could hardly be expressed in terms of all or none homology since there might exist variable degrees of homology and pairing. Here it may be noted that much too less pairing within *Secale* genome was observed by these workers than that expected on the basis of LEVAN'S (1942) findings in haploid rye. It may be that genotypic conditions regarding the control of synapsis in these materials are not at all comparable.

4. With Hordeum.

QUINCKE (1940) reported failure of his attempt to cross *Hordeum vulgare* and *Secale cereale*. The zygote failed to develop further within a short time after fertilization. On the other hand, BRINK *et al* (1944) and COOPER and BRINK (1944) easily succeeded in making crosses between *Hordeum jubatum* (♀ parent) and *Secale cereale* (♂ parent). The reciprocal cross was not attempted. They found that hybrid embryos ceased to grow after 6 to 13 days after fertilization and by culturing them in vitro it could be shown that this collapse was basically due to the failure of endosperm to turn cellular like in normal plants thus antipodals remaining retarded (this type of sterility is termed as somatoplastic). One hybrid individual was however grown to maturity and it showed intermediacy with respect to growth habit, high sterility and at diakinesis 5 II + 7 I. At anaphase nondisjunctive tendency seemed to give rise to bridges. In another study by BRINK and COOPER (1944), *Hordeum vulgare* was used as seed parent. In this case the antipodals did not show any division, the endosperm also failing in same way and hybrids died even earlier than in case of *H. jubatum*.

In striking contrast to above, THOMPSON (1939, 1940) and THOMPSON and JOHNSTON (1945) observed none of these irregularities in the hybrids between *H. hexastichum* and *S. cereale*, although they found endosperm nuclei to be fewer, larger in size and coenocytic. Embryos died after four days. SMITH (1942) also did not succeed in crosses using *H. bulbosum*.

5. With Haynaldia.

In an attempt to transfer extreme hardiness and drought resistance from *Haynaldia hordeacea* to *cereale* rye, ZHUKOVSKY (1944) obtained a fertile hybrid between them, using *Haynaldia* parent as pollen source. NAKAJIMA (1951, 1953) used *H. villosa* as the seed parent and in hybrid he observed at M I 0–2 bivalents and 10–14 univalents. On backcrossing to rye 12 segregants resembling rye and with 2n = 20, 21 resulted and showed high sterility. The author also believed some heterogenetic pairing to have occurred. Trigeneric hybrids like (*Triticum dicoccum* × *Haynaldia villosa*) × *S. cereale* were reported by KOSTOFF (1936) and NAKAJIMA (1952).

II. GENETICS

FRUWIRTH (1923) and MATSUURA (1933) included rye in their comprehensive monographs and therefore a useful summary of genetic studies on record prior to 1929 can be found in these two references. Unfortunately, even till this day the genetics of this important genus has not received much attention therefore not to mention the linkage groups even simple markers so often needed in any cytogenetic research have not been identified sufficiently. A few characters are discussed below under individual heads while others have been summarized in Table 9 (see later, p. 427).

1. Periodicity.

TSCHERMAK (1906) was studying the interspecific hybrid between *S. montanum*, a perennial, and *S. cereale*, an annual or sometimes biennial and he found perennial habit to be dominant. It should be pointed out here that this cross has been severally investigated in the past for transferring the perennial character from *montanum* parent to *cereale* strains. The dominance of perenniality were also noted by DERZHAVIN (1935) and KRASNJUK (1935) who were using *Kuprijanovii* × *cereale* and wheat × rye hybrids respectively. PRICE (1955) in F_1 of *cereale* × *montanum* and STUTZ (1957) in F_2 observed that flowering time greatly varied and some plants tended to flower in the next growing season which however, can not be used as a criterion of perennial habit. OSSENT (1930) reported from his study of this same hybrid, that F_1's perished at second or third harvest while F_2's gave a variable population thus indicating that perenniality is only incompletely dominant over annual habit. DUKA (1935) on the other hand believed that perenniality behaved as recessive. Thus it seems to be showing a variable degree of dominance which is not surprising in view of HARLAND's (1936) findings in the species crosses of genus *Gossypium*, STUTZ's (1957) interpretation of his data on the elymoides mutant in rye and the theoretical work by R. A. FISHER and others on the evolution of dominance. The perennial character has great value to the plant breeder and therefore its genetics should be investigated in more detail.

2. Rachis fragility.

The fragile character of species while of selective value for the seed dispersal in wild species, is undesirable from the farmer's viewpoint. Also this character has been used by several workers in classification. That fragility is dominant over toughness has been verified by several authors. TSCHERMAK (1906 and later), DERZHAVIN (1935), OSSENT (1930), and KOSTOFF (1937) reported some evidence in interspecific as well as intraspecific crosses whereas ANTROPOV (unpub., cited after KARPECHENKO et al, 1929) studied the intergeneric hybrid *Secale cereale* × *Aegilops* spp., the rye being male parent and with tough rachis character. Except for the dominance situation, no data on the nature of segregation or genetic ratios seem to have been recorded.

3. 'Hairy-neck' character (i.e. pubescence of peduncle.)

It was mentioned earlier that the hairy neck character of rye serves as a good phenotypic marker in the studies on wheat-rye hybrid. TSCHERMAK (1906) found pubescence to be dominant over the glabrousness in a cross between *cereale* and *montanum*. Later LEIGHTY and TAYLOR (1924) observed in the progeny of naturally occurring wheat-rye hybrids a highly irregular segregation for hairy-neck (HN) and they could select three wheat-like groups (designated as C,H and K respectively) that on being crossed to wheat parent gave in F_2 about 25%, 62.9% and 36.2% plants with hairy-neck. No explanation for these ratios was attempted. However, the possibility of such a gene transfer from one genus to another has aroused considerable interest in HN character as indicated by several authors (for instance, LOVE and CRAIG, 1919; FLORELL, 1931; OEHLER 1938; TAYLOR, 1934; KATTERMANN, 1937 and later; LEDINGHAM and THOMPSON, 1938). O'MARA (1953) points out its frequent mention in Russian literature.

The study of TAYLOR (1934) merits special mention. He found that HN behaved as dominant in the F_1 generation but subsequently very irregularly, or even as a recessive to smooth peduncle. He assumed for a marked deficiency of HN segregates among the backcrosses to wheat

that about 10% of the gametes carrying HN-factor were being eliminated and also possibly some loss of HN at somatic mitoses took place.
However, O'MARA (1951) disfavored his suggestion of those backcross
products with HN being 'disomic additions' to wheat genome. Recently JONES and JENSEN (1954) have studied two sets of wheat-rye
crosses and found HN to be inherited on monofactorical basis (the F_2
had 73.8% and 74.0% HN plants respectively). According to these
authors, the transfer could take place in two ways namely (1) by
substitution of a chromosome pair of wheat by that of rye, or (2)
through reciprocal translocation between the two complements. It is
difficult to see how any of these unusual events can occur so regularly
and further investigations are to be awaited on this issue.

Some evidence is available for a genetic association between the
hairy-neck character and reduction in fertility (FLORELL, 1931;
KATTERMANN, 1937), higher tillering (TAYLOR 1934) and shorter culms
(OEHLER, 1938; O'MARA, 1951).

4. Seed colour and size: cases of xenia.

In 1893 GILTAY first reported xenia in rye with reference to seed
colour (the term xenia signifies direct observable effect of the
genetic constitution of pollen on the zygote). RÜMKER (1911, 1912)
was able to obtain pure 'races' for an array of aleurone colours. viz
deep blue, greenish blue to yellow and deep brown. Also he noted the
seeds of the cross yellow ♀ × green ♂ to have yellow grains with
green tinge, and in F_2 3 green: 1 yellow. STEGLEICH and PIPER
(1922) carefully analysed their observations to show that colour
of aleurone and epidermis (outer coat) were inherited independently
of each other. They concluded that bluish aleurone colour was
dominant to colorless and so also black coat colour to white.
DUMON (1938) on the other hand reported in F_1 of a cross yellow ♀ ×
brown ♂ green grain colour and in F_2 the dihybrid ratio 9 green:
3 brown: 4 yellow so that he assumed the interaction of two factors
as follows: AAbb-brown, aaBB-yellow and AABB-green. DUMON
also observed other dominance relationships in another cross. In
order to study various combinations of the colours in pericarp,
testa and aleurone layers, NEUMANN and PELSHENKE (1954) constructed the following useful chart:

TABLE 6. Grain colour chart (After NEUMANN-PELSHENKE, 1954).

Colour of grain	Pericarp	Testa	Aleurone
Green	Greyish yellow as basic tint	Yellow to yellow brown	Blue
Dry-green	,,	Weak yellow	Blue
Yellow	,,	Yellow	Yellow or noncoloured
Blue	Membranous	,,	Weak blue
Silver grey or greyish yellow	Thick opaque	,,	,,

As for seed size inheritance, NICOLAISEN (1932) believed it to be another case of xenia whereas FRIMMEL (1939) and WELLENSIEK (1948) have reported evidence of maternal inheritance (cytoplasmic?).

5. Partial sterility (Schartigkeit).

The widespread occurrence of partial sterility in many cultivated strains and its importance as a problem for plant breeders was clearly recognized by ÜLRICH (1902) who found average seedset in three German varieties- Petkus, Probsteier and Schlanstedter- to be about 78%, 61% and 79% respectively. LANDES (1939) was inclined to attribute this to irregularities in the development of endosperm. PLÄHN (1927) and HAUPT (1928) first pointed out that partial sterility was inherited. The papers by LEITH (1925) and SHANDS (1938) reported some data in American strains in which some amount of structural heterozygosity was present and might be an important cause of poor seedsetting. MÜNTZING (1946b) found a significant parent-offspring correlation in his material where both cytological and genetical causes were present. It was mentioned earlier that 'Tetra-rye' shows even greater degrees of partial sterility.

6. Pollen sterility.

DAVIDSON et al (1924) reported rather frequent rise of pollen sterile individuals among inbred rye populations. However, these workers did not analyse for heritable, monogenic cases. MÜNTZING (1939) classified as many as 50% plants in a population of 610 plants under observation to be pollen steriles. Careful investigations by PUTT (1954) showed a

lack of correlation with cytological irregulatities that are fairly com-
monplace in rye populations. He crossed low × high pollen sterile
plants and found F_1 progenies to be more fertile thus indicating pollen
sterility to behave as recessive. Furthermore in F_2, F_3 and F_4 generations of a cross between two inbreds, he obtained evidence of cytoplasmic inheritance of pollen abortion independently from ovular
sterility. Finally he concluded this character to have a rather complex
basis of inheritance involving several dominant and recessive factors
as well as the control by cytoplasm.

7. Self-incompatibility.

Examples of both inbreeding and outbreeding systems occur among
the members of *Secale* genus. *S. africanum*, *S. sylvestre*, and *S. vavilovii*,
for instance, are self-compatible, the last one tending to be cleistoga-
mous; *cereale* and all members of *montanum-Kuprijanovii* complex
seem to possess self-incompatibility systems. The discussion to be
given here is entirely for *cereale* since others do not seem to be investigated as yet. In 1907, JOHST reported that in self-incompatible pollinations, pollen tube failed to grow after certain stage. However,
contrary to his results, incompatibility in rye has not been found to be
absolute. Different varieties and plants within a variety may differ in
the ability to set seed upon selfing, the average being in the range of
1–10% and the ratio of open/self seed set being about 10–50 (LUND-
QVIST, 1958b). It is significant to note that these differences are largely
heritable and the self seeding ability may be increased by selection. In
general, rye is relatively less susceptible to inbreeding deterioration
than corn and several other outbreeding crop species.

Although most investigators seem to have primarily a practical aim
in its study, the genetics of self-incompatibility in rye is being under-
stood, notably due to the brilliant researches by LUNDQVIST (1947 et
seq.). HERIBERT-NILSSON (1916) first reported this character to be
monogenic, recessive and later (1953) found that several factors might
be involved. The results of BREWBAKER (1926) were also not explicable
on basis of any simple genetic scheme and the genotype-environment
interactions seemed to be predominant. That self-compatibility
behaves as a dominant in crosses between high and low compatible
lines has been severally reported (for instance, PETERSON (1934; KRAS-
NJUK, 1936) but as LUNDQVIST (1958b) points out, without a knowledge

of the incompatibility system, no adequate interpretation could be possible. HERIBERT-NILSSON (1953) also noted the majority of high-seeding individuals in segregating generations and he postulated a minimum of two polymeric factors for self-compatibility.

Results of LUNDQVIST'S (1954, 1956, 1957, 1958a, b) studies are summarized here and the reader may consult original publications for details and better insight into this subject. In rye, (a) this character is gametophytically controlled by two independent, multiallelic loci (the presence of modifying factors was nonetheless indicated); (b) both factors of the pollen have to be matched in the style for incompatible reaction; so that these two factors seem to cooperate in producing these specificities; and (c) this may have a direct bearing on the persistence of self-incompatibility at the tetraploid level. Reviewing the known examples of one-locus, gametophytic system, LUNDQVIST points out the fundamental difference between these systems.

Both S and Z loci are capable of mutations rendering the haploid pollen compatible in the self style. The occurrence of such mutant self-compatible plants was earlier indicated in the works of BREWBAKER (1926), AGEEW (1929), PETERSON (1934) and HERIBERT-NILSSON (1953). The Z locus has given some evidence of a compound structure with pollen- and stylar-active parts. Unlike the onelocus system of, say, *Nicotiana*, which enforces obligate heterozygosity, here evidence from comparison of heterozygous-heterozygous with siblings having heterozygous-hemozygous combination at these loci shows that homozygosity for these chromosome regions did not bring a deleterious effect on viability or vegetative growth (LUNDQVIST, 1958a).

One important aspect of this character is its behaviour in successive selfed generations. Table 7 gives a comparison of some data reported

TABLE 7. Data on self-sterility.

Author: Material:	AGEEW (1929) Vjatka rye		BREWBAKER (1926) Minnesota 2.		PETERSON (1934) Minnesota 2.		MENGERSEN (1951) Petkus	
Data:	Gen.	%setting	Gen.	%setting	Gen.	%setting	Gen.	%setting
	S_1	0.0	S_1	3.1	S_3	4.8	S_1	14.2
	S_2	8.4	S_2	4.7	S_5	19.7	S_2	33.1
	S_3	33.7	S_3	9.1	S_6	29.1	S_3	41.7
			S_4	14.1	S_7	43.1	S_{15}-S_{20}	47.1
			S_5	7.7	S_8	46.6		

by AGEEW (1929), BREWBAKER (1926), PETERSON (1934) and MEN-
GERSEN (1950, 1951). It is evidently clear that self-seeding ability in
general increased with progressive inbreeding. However, LUNDQVIST
(1958b) concludes that "up to about 25% seedset in parents, the offspring mean as a rule exceeds its parental class value ... the causes of
low offspring seed set may be different for the two parental categories
(low and high seeding)". The parent-offspring correlations in his diploid and tetraploid populations were all positive and significant
(Table 8).

TABLE 8. Parent-offspring correlations for self-seeding ability
(LUNDQVIST, 1958b).

Culture	Diploids			Tetraploids		
	46/47	47/48	48/49	46/47	47/48	48/49
Pop./S_1	0.874	0.301	0.363	0.380	0.385	0.136
S_1/S_2	0.707	0.672	0.680	0.352	0.534	0.601
S_2/S_3	—	0.449	0.645	—	0.180	0.446

It should be noted here that in the inbred derivatives of tetraploid
populations, he noted pronounced skewness towards low-seeding for
practically all parental types. As compared to the diploids, there was
increased variability both between years and between generations.
Data of LÖWENSTEIN (1951) and PLARRE (1954) on self-incompatibility
in tetraploids seem to agree in general with above.

8. Winter versus spring growth habit.

From his studies of a cross Heinreich (winter rye) × Sachsischen
Standen (spring rye), TSCHERMAK (1906) concluded that spring habit
was dominant and found in F_2 a 3 : 1 ratio if spring form was used as
the mother parent and a 4.6 (spring) : 1 (winter form) ratio in its
reciprocal. Later PURVIS (1939) using both forms derived from Petkus
rye showed that in flowering, tillering and lack of response to vernalization, the hybrids closely resembled the spring parent but in following
generation (i.e. F_2) she did not get such a discrete and discontinous
variation indicating that perhaps several genes were governing this
character and each one associated with different degree of earliness
effect. She further assumed that since vernalization and various other
treatments could modify both the winter and late maturing characters,

the 'spring' gene might simulate in its physiological effect to that for earliness. A few papers may be found on the subject of this conversion from one habit to another (for instance, STUBBE ,1955).

9. *Disease and pest resistance.*

Most investigations on the disease and insect pest resistance in rye seem to be only casual field observations. SORAUER in 1909 listed eight German varieties that were found to be susceptible to rusts. That resistance to leaf rust (*Puccinia dispersa*) is a heritable character seems to be recognized from early times (ROEMER, 1939). ERIKSSON (1921) published a monograph on all known fungous diseases and in it he reports Petkus rye to be immune or highly resistant to the snow mold. LEVINE and STAKMAN (1923) investigated the causal organism of stem rust *Puccinia graminis secalis*, from the viewpoint of its biological specialization and the susceptibility of three common varieties (Rosen, Prolific and Swedish).The inheritance of resistance to leaf rust was first analysed by MAINS and LEIGHTY (1923) who made crosses between individuals with high and low resistance and found the resistance to be dominant over susceptibility, however controlled by a multifactorial complex. Among the progeny of highly resistant combinations selfed as well as intercrossed with each other, MAINS (1926) recovered a wide array of reaction levels with respect to stem and leaf rusts and powdery mildew (*Erysiphe graminis secalis*), in a range from nearly complete immunity to rather high susceptibility. Thus although a genic analysis did not seem possible from his data, it appeared evident that in each case resistance was dominant and that it was inherited on independent basis for three different pathogens. Further, inspite of fairly high amount of self-sterility in his material, MAINS (1926) succeeded in producing a strain true breeding for resistance to all three diseases mentioned above after three generations of selfing followed by selection. GARBINI (1950) reported the Massaux-hybrid strains developed in Pergamino to be having high degrees of resistance to leaf rust. CZARNOKA (1939) earlier mentioned a Polish rye variety to be resistant to stem rust and such instances are also found among primitive rye and *Secale montanum*.

The genetics of resistance to Sclerotic disease, also known as 'Mutterkorn' (*Claviceps purpurea*) and stone blight has not been investigated so far (WARMBRUNN, 1952). MOTHES and SILBER (1952) found the

Mutterkorn disease developing more often on the sterile or unfertilized florets. *Urocystis occulta* causes the stem blight which is easily controlled by cauterization and therefore has not been a problem for plant breeders.

In many regions of Belgium, Denmark, England and USSR (GOF-FART, 1951) and also Netherlands (DEWEZ, 1950), eelworm (*Ditylenchus dipsaci*) causes considerable damage to rye crop. KOTTHOFF (1942) reported some of the agricultural strains in Netherlands to have resistance or tolerance. WELLENSIEK (1945, 1947) studied the cross Ottersumer × Petkus rye and found resistance to behave as dominant over susceptibliity.

10. Anomalous mutants.

Among their inbred material, DAVIDSON *et al* (1924) noted the occurrence of a few plants with brittle stems. In F_2 of a cross between normal and mutant individuals, they obtained 98 normal: 26 brittle-stem indicating the mutation to be recessive. Further studies with this mutation have shown the brittle-stem individuals to differ from normal ones by their higher pentosan and colloidal content and lower lignin as well as crude fiber content (DAVIDSON *et al*, 1924), thinner cell wall (BREWBAKER, 1926), a reduction in sclerenchyma of vascular bundles (LADA, 1933) and by a lower percentage of silicic acid (HORNBURG, 1929).

HERIBERT-NILSSON (1913) found in the progeny of an intravarietal cross a typical case of variegation represented by yellow and white (albino) seedlings. This albinism was shown to be a monogenic recessive character (HERIBERT-NILSSON, 1913; KALT, 1916). DAVIDSON *et al* (1924) seemed to believe that such albinos occur as frequently as 35% individuals among some inbred strains and even more than 50% among the strains derived by bulk selection. From a sample of seeds of *S. anatolicum* and of *cereale* var. elymoides (to be described below) the present writer obtained 6% and 9.4% plants respectively showing various degrees of albinism and variegation patterns, and unfortunately none of these survived after two or three leaf stage. A few cases had soon recovered the normal appearance and were found to be genetically also perfectly normal.

SIRKS (1929) described an unusual type of chlorophyll deficiency which he termed as 'Lichtempfindlichkeit' (i.e. light sensitivity). Certain individuals in a strain of rye seemed to have chlorophyll destroyed by too intensive sunlight thus appearing with partially white glumes, and when subjected to insolation and low night temperatures (about 2°C), were observed to lose chlorophyll entirely eventually turning brown and this sensitivity he found to behave as a monogenic recessive condition (F_2 ratio 283 unaltered: 101 altered). From a different strain a corresponding ratio of 161 : 7 was obtained.

DUMON and LAEREMANS (1957) assumed two factors A_1-a_1, A_2-a_2 for the control of production of anthocyanin in plants of virescent type, such that A_1 is dominant to A_2, and $A_1A_1a_2a_2WW$, $a_1a_1a_2a_2WW$ give pinkish yellow and canary yellow colours respectively.

BREWBAKER (1926) described some more cases of chlorophyll deficiency of which a yellow-green striped type appeared to be much variable in colour pattern whereas another golden-green blend type tended to have a much deeper, uniform yellowish colour with yellow and green stripes intermingled together. On the other hand, a third type, socalled virescent-white, turned gradually into yellowish-green and eventually normal green when placed under usual growth conditions. BREWBAKER found each one to behave as a monofactorial, recessive condition.

THOMPSON (1922) reported the occurrence of plants with branched ears and he called them 'Alaska types'. VAVILOV (1925) found several of them in his collections of cultivated rye and placed them under a new variety, *S. cereale* var. *monstrosum*. SMAGIN (1940) was led to conclude from his observations that the frequency of branched ears progressively increased as one grew progeny of such ears each time and BROJOVIC (1953) showed the condition to be inherited. On the contrary, a host of papers have been appearing in Russian literature that report how certain growth conditions such as high level of fertilizer application, short photoperiod or vernalization can induce this branching of ears in rye. An attempt to induce it by irradiating germinating seeds however failed completely (LEKEZYNSKA and WIONECK, 1954). Some workers have pointed out its potential value in practical farming and the method of applying higher nutrient doses has been suggested (ROD and VRZEVSKII, 1954, and VRESKY, 1955, for instance).

The elymoides mutant reported by STUTZ (1958) had three spikelets instead of one at a node and some of the mutant segregates obtained in subsequent generations had variable numbers of spikelets at a

TABLE 9. Summary of other genetic data.

Character	Material used (type of crosses)	Inheritance dom. rec.	Reference
Maturity	Interspecific	Earliness vs. lateness	TSCHERMAK (1906)
Germinability	,,	Late vs. early	,,
Growth vigour	Intravarietal	High vs. poor: variable	KRESS (1938)
Growth habit	Interspecific	Erect vs. prostrate	OSSENT (1930, 1938)
Coleoptile colour	—	Greenish grains giving red coleoptile dominant over yellow grain giving reddish coleoptile.	DUMON (1938, 1957)
		Red vs. green	TREBOUX (1925)
Culm height	Intervarietal	Long vs. short (1 : 2 : 1)	TSCHERMAK (1906)
	Intervarietal	Long vs. short (3 : 1)	KRASNJUK (1936)
Stem and leaf glaucousness	Interspecific	Glaucous vs. smooth	TSCHERMAK (1906)
,,	,,	,,	HERIBERT-NILSSON (1917)
Leaf sheath pubescence	Interspecific	Pubescent vs. glabrous	TSCHERMAK (1906)
Ligule	Intervarietal	Presence vs. absence	KRASNJUK (1936)
Auricle colour	Interspecific	Red vs. green	TSCHERMAK (1906)
Ear shape	Intervarietal	Long, narrow vs. short, broad.	FRIMMEL and BARANEK (1935)
Ear density	Intervarietal	Dense vs. lax	TSCHERMAK (1906)
Awning	Intergeneric	Awned vs. awnless	KARPECHENKO (1929)
Glume pubescence	Interspecific	Pubescent vs. smooth	TSCHERMAK (1906)
Seed size	Intervarietal	Large vs. small	,,
,,	Interspecific	,,	OSSENT (1930)

node which is a characteristic met with in the genus *Elymus* and be-haved as a simple recessive, the segregation in F_2 being 3 : 1 although various other ratios also occurred showing differences in respect to both penetrance and expressivity. For instance, in an F_2 from ely-moides $\times$ *S. montanum* a ratio of 79 mutant : 31 normal was obtained which this author considered to have involved penetrance effect.

In Table 9 above are listed inheritance studies on some other characters than those mentioned already and it should be pointed out that in almost all instances, a monofactorial ratio (either 3 : 1 or 1 : 2 : 1 in F_2) has been reported. It will be apparent that relatively very little work has been done in rye genetics and that also with the material including wheat-rye hybrids and *cereale* $\times$ *montanum* hybrids. In the opinion of this writer, the former due to the fact that wheat and rye chromosomes do not pair and are nonhomologous and the latter for the presence of possibly specific modifier complexes (a situation so well explored in *Gossypium* by S. C. HARLAND and others) may not be suitable material to use in such inheritance studies. That rye has a self-incompatibility system, makes it perhaps difficult to obtain sufficiently large numbers of nearly homozygous families but in this context a method suggested by forage crop breeders could be considered here. Accordingly, instead of requiring homozygous material, different F_1 plants may be analysed separately and instead of using F_2 or F_3, relatively large backcross families be obtained by handpollination. Moreover, as pointed out earlier, self-fertility in rye is subject to improvement and desirable inbred lines can be developed.

III. SYSTEMATICS

The genus *Secale*, a member of Tribe Hordeae, is relatively very small but the number of 'good' species recognized and the basis of their classification are not unequivocally known as yet. KÖRNICKE (1885) considered a single species, *cereale*, and recognized its four varieties on basis of ear colour and shape. The socalled two-species system was perhaps initiated by ASCHERSON and GRAEBNER (1901) who mentioned *sylvestre*, an annual with completely fragile rachis, and *cereale*- annual, cultivated and with tough rachis. VAVILOV (1917, 1925) collected during his famous expeditions an enormous amount of material and he had recognized four species, namely *cereale* (further classifying into 24 botanical varieties), *montanum*, *africanum* and *fragile* (synonymous with *sylvestre*, as severally pointed out by E. SCHIEMANN) on the basis of both vegetative and ear characters. Figure 14 shows the distribution of these species as given by VAVILOV (1925), and the supposed two centers of origin. GROSSHEIM (1924) first described *vavilovii*, an annual wild species, recently shown to be having a tendency towards cleistogamy (KRANZ, 1957). It may also be mentioned here that SCHIEMANN (1932, 1948) placed *vavilovii* under either *fragile*, or possibly *montanum*. The classification given by her is briefly as follows:

I. Section Agrestes.

    1. *Secale sylvestre* Host. (syn. *fragile*).
    2.   ,,   *montanum* Guss.
    3.   ,,   *africanum* Stapf.

II. Section Cerealia.

    4. *Secale ancestrale* Zhuk.
    5.   ,,   *cereale* L.

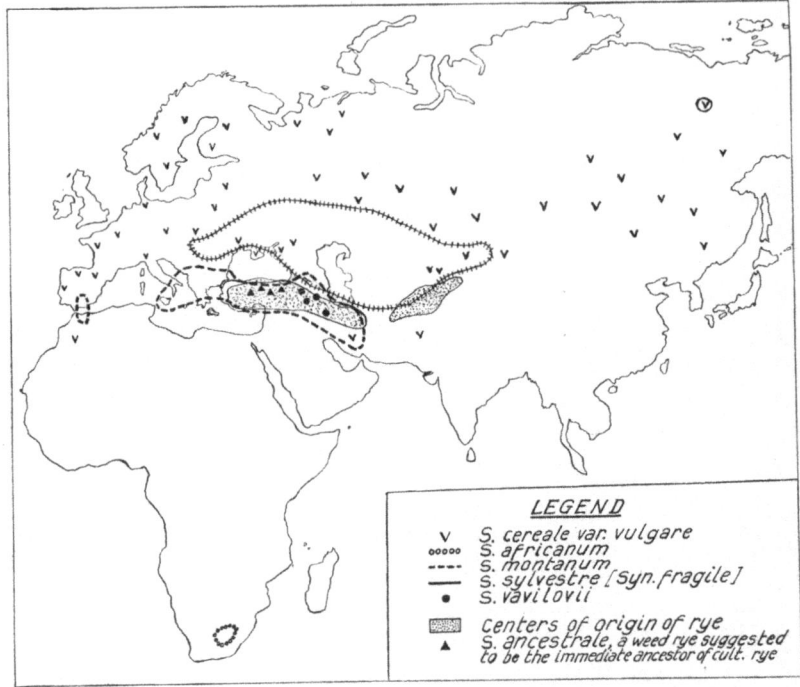

Fig. 14. Map showing distribution of some *Secale* species. (adapted after VAVILOV, 1925).

ROSHEVITZ (1948) as a 'splitter' on the other hand, recognized as many as 14 different species under three sections as below:

I. Section Silvestria.
    Annual, wild, fragile rachis, Includes only *sylvestre*.

II. Section Kuprijanovia.
    Perennial, with short rhizomes and fragile rachis (except *daralgessi* that has tough rachis). Includes *Kuprijanovii*, *ciliatoglume*, *dalmaticum*, *montanum*, *anatolicum*, *africanum* and *daralgessi*.

III. Section Cerealia.
    Annual but rarely biennial also and rachis fragile (except for the cultivated *cereale* rye). Includes *vavilovii*, *ancestrale*, *afghanicum*, *dighoricum*, *segetale* and *cereale*.

It might be recalled that cytological study of interspecific hybrids has shown *vavilovii* as having the same chromosome arrangement as *montanum* and *africanum* so that it is suggested that these should be placed together in same section. The Transcaucasian strain, incorrectly named as *vavilovii*, has been shown to have the *cereale*-type of chromosome arrangement and morphologically seems to agree with the description of *segetale*, as given by ROSHEVITZ (1948). Thus in this review, only five species (Figure 13) have been dealt with whereas *anatolicum*, *dalmaticum* and *Kuprijanovii*, to follow STUTZ (1957), were considered as if they belong to a Rassenkreis, the *montanum* group. Similarly, it may be that *afghanicum*, *dighoricum* and *segetale* are only ecotypes, or microgeographic races, of cereale. The case of *ancestrale*, a weed rye, also needs to be investigated especially because it is generally regarded as the immediate ancestor of cultivated rye.

IV. ORIGIN OF CULTIVATED RYE

Previously it was mentioned that from his systematic study of various collections VAVILOV (1917, et. seq.) established two main regions of diversity. These are: (1) Afghanistan, Bokhara and Eastern Persia, and (2) Armenia, Georgia, Asia Minor and S.W. Persia (Fig. 14). Later, extensive work by GROSSHEIM (1924) and his associates, on collections from Transcaucasia, by BERKNER and MEYER (1927), SCHEIBE (1935) and POPOFF (1939) on those from Turkey, Anatolia and Bulgaria respectively gave strong support to VAVILOV's conclusions. Thus rye as a cultivated plant seems to be of no importance in its geographical centers of origin. According to VAVILOV, some weedy rye of barley and wheat fields in Orient had given rise to cultivated rye through domestication and selection. This hypothesis stimulated a search for weedy ancestor and in 1928, ZHUKOVSKY described an endemic form of West Anatolia under the name, *Secale ancestrale*. SCHIEMANN (1932, and later) joined this viewpoint. ROSHEVITZ (1948) further suggested that section Cerealia includes a number of weedy forms such as *afghanicum, segetale, dighoricum* and *ancestrale*, and these were possibly derived from *vavilovii*. However, in light of recent cytological studies, this view seems to be no more tenable.

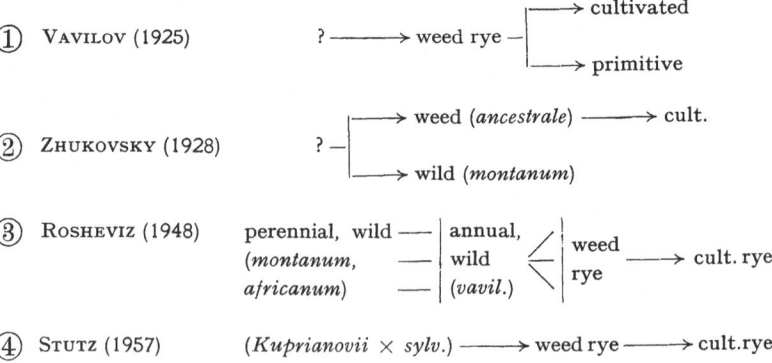

STUTZ (1957), on the other hand, argued in favour of a hybrid origin of weedy ancestor of cultivated rye. Accordingly, these weedy pioneers having hardiness and vigour of perennial types combined with annual habit originated from among the products of hybridization between *sylvestre* and some member of the Kuprijanovii section. KRANZ (1957) also held the opinion that a few characters of Iranian primitive rye like three florets per spikelet and red auricular joint possibly came from *sylvestre* and *montanum* respectively, and likewise the two observed translocation patterns might have been derived from some ancient representative of the genus (viz. *sylvestre*) that on splitting under certain favorable environmental conditions fortuitously fixed two potentially new lines presumably through their effectiveness as linked adaptive complexes. As pointed out by STEBBINS (1950, p. 247), "the most valuable evidence which could be secured in favour of this hypothesis would be the demonstration of the existence of chromosomal types with differential selective values in a species population which appeared to be in the process of breaking up". Furthermore, one would have to obtain F_1 and subsequent progenies on a large scale for being able to recover types approximating those segregants which were originally acted upon by natural selection.

Finally, it seems necessary to emphasize that along with structural alterations of chromosomes, the role of genetic differentiation in speciation processes appears to merit considerable attention by rye workers since both these sets of evolutionary changes are complementary rather than mutually exclusive. KRANZ (1957) points out that *Secale* is an actively expanding genus and it may be hoped that evolutionary research offers great promise and interest.

REFERENCES

AASE, H. C., 1930. Cytology of hybrids. Res. Stud. State Coll. Wash. 2: 1–60.

AASE, H. C., 1935. Cytology of cereals. I. Bot. Rev. 1: 467–96.

AASE, H. C., 1946. Cytology of cereals. II. Bot. Rev. 12: 255–34.

AASE, H. C. and L. POWERS, 1926. Chromosome numbers in crop plants. Amer. Journ. Bot. 13: 367–72.

AGEEW, K. F., 1929. (Inbreeding in rye). Arb. Landw. Timirj. Akad. Mosk. 4: 143–74.

AKDIK, S. and A. MÜNTZING, 1949. New cases of segmental interchanges and some other meiotic peculiarities in rye. Hereditas 35: 67–76.

ANTONOFF, S., 1936. Beitrag zum zytogenetischen Studium der Artbastarde *Triticum turgidum* × *T. durum* and *Secale cereale* × *S. montanum*. Züchter 8: 240–43.

ANTROPOV, V. and V., 1936. (Flora of cultivated plants, Rye). Leningr. Akad.

BACKHOUSE, W. O., 1916. Note on the inheritance of crossability. Journ. Genet. 6: 91–94.

BELLING, J., 1925. Fracture of chromosome in rye. Journ. Hered. 16: 360.

BERG, K. H., 1931. Autosyndese in *Aegilops triuncialis* L. × *Secale cereale* L. Zschr. Pflanzenz: 17: 55–69.

BLEIER, H., 1930. Cytologie von Art- und Gattungbastarden des Getreides. Züchter 2: 12–22.

BLEIER, H., 1950. Genommutation als neue praktische Zuchtmethode. DLG-Nachr. Pflanzenz. Wiesbaden.

BOROJEVIC, S., 1953. (Branched ears in rye, *Secale cereale*). Poljopr. Znanst. Smot. 15: 75–87.

BOSE, S., 1956. Aberrations in the nucleolar chromosome of inbred rye. Hereditas 42: 263–92.

BOSEMARK, N. O., 1957. Further studies on accessory chromosomes in grasses. Hereditas 43: 236–97.

BRADLEY, M. V., 1948. A method of making acetocarmine squashes permanent without removal of the coverslip. Stain Techn. 23: 41–44.

BRAGDO, M., 1955. Production of polyploids by colchicine. Euphytica 4: 76–82.

BRAVO, A. R., 1956. (The efficiency of lindane as an agent for inducing polyploidy in rye). Acta Agron. Palmeria 6: 143–47.

BREMER, G. and D. E. BREMER-REINDERS, 1954. Breeding of tetraploid rye in the Netherlands. I. Methods and cytological investigations. Euphytica 3: 49–63.

BREMER-REINDERS, D. E. and G. BREMER, 1952. Methods used for producing polyploid agricultural plants. Euphytica 1: 87–94.

BRESLAVETZ, L., 1939. Polyploids in rye induced by X-rays. Compt. Rend. (Dokl.) Akad. Sci. URSS 22: 354–57.

BRESLAVETZ, L. P., 1940. Polyploid forms of spring rye. Compt. Rend. (Dokl.) Akad. Sci. URSS 29: 328–31.

BRESLAVETZ, L. P., G. B. MEDWEDEWA and A. S. AFANASJEWA, 1935. Die Wirkung der Röntgenstrahlen auf Roggen. Protoplasma 23: 520–33.

BREWBAKER, H. E., 1926. Studies of self-fertilization in rye. Minn. A. E. S. Techn. Bull. 40: 40 pp.

BRINK, R. A. and D. C. COOPER, 1944. The antipodals in relation to abnormal endosperm behaviour in *Hordeum jubatum* × *Secale cereale* hybrid seeds. Genetics 29: 391–406.

BRINK, R. A., D. C. COOPER and L. E. AUSHERMAN, 1944. A hybrid between *Hordeum jubatum* and *Secale cereale*. Journ. Hered. 35: 67–75.

BUCHINGER, A., 1931. Ein Roggen-Weizen und Weizen-Roggen Bastard. Züchter 3: 329–33.

BUCHINGER, A., 1933. Zur Genetik der *Aegilops-Weizen* und *Aegilops-Roggen* Bastarde. Genetica 15: 299–342.

CHAPMAN, V. and R. RILEY, 1955. The disomic addition of rye chromosome II to wheat. Nature 175: 1091.

CHIN, J. C., 1943. Cytology of the autotetraploid rye. Bot. Gaz. 104: 627–32.

COOPER, D. C. and R. A. BRINK, 1944. Collapse of the seed following the mating of *Hordeum jubatum* × *Secale cereale*. Genetics 29: 370–90.

CZARNOCKA, J., 1939. Zyto Pulawskie wezesne i metodj gigo hodowli. Bibl. Pulawska 20: 29.

DARLINGTON, C. D., 1933. The origin and behaviour of chiasmata. VIII. *Secale cereale*. Cytologia 4: 444–52.

DARLINGTON, C. D., 1937. Recent advances in cytology. 2nd ed. Blakiston.

DARLINGTON, C. D. and L. F. LACOUR, 1940. Nucleic acid starvation of chromosomes in *Trillium*. Journ. Genet. 40: 185–213.

DARLINGTON, C. D. and A. P. WYLIE, 1956. Chromosome atlas of flowering plants.

DAVIDSON, F. R., H. E. BREWBAKER and N. A. THOMPSON, 1924. Brittle-straw and other abnormalities in rye. Journ. Agric. Res. 28: 169–72.

DERZHAVIN, A. I., 1935. (Further data on the perennial rye, *Secale Kuprijanovii* Gross. and its agricultural value). Bull. Appl. Bot. Ser. A: 14: 159–65.

DEWEZ, W., 1940. Het optreden van het stengelaaltje (*Tylenchus dipsaci*) in Limburg. Tijdschr. Plantenz. 46: 194–204.

DOBZHANSKY, TH., 1951. Genetics and the origin of species. 3rd. ed. Columbia.

DOLGUSIN, D. A., 1953. (An experiment on producing rye from an oat plant). Agrobiologija 5: 86–91.

DORSEY, E., 1936. Induced polyploidy in wheat and rye. Journ. Hered. 27: 155–60.

DUKA, S. KH., 1935. Cytogenetic research on the interspecific hybrid *Secale cereale* × *S. montanum*. Bull. Appl. Bot. Ser/A. 14: 233–38.

DUMON, A. G., 1938. (A case of dominant and recessive brown in *Secale cereale*). (French) Agric. Louvain 41: 190–96.

DUMON, A. G. and R. LAEREMANS, 1957. Contribution à l'analyse génétique de l'anthocyane du siègle. Bull. Jard. bot. Brux. 27: 507–13.

ELLERSTRÖM, S. and A. HÅGBERG, 1954. Competition between diploids and tetraploids in mixed rye populations. Hereditas 40: 535–37.

EMME, H., 1927. Zur Cytologie der Gattung *Secale* L. Bull. Appl. Bot. 17: 73–100.

EMME, H., 1928. Karyologie der Gattung *Secale* L. Zschr. ind. Abst. Vererb. L. 47: 99–124.

ERIKSSON, J., 1912. (Fungoid diseases of agricultural plants). Translated by A. MOLANDER, 208 pp.

FERRAND, A., 1923. Note sur la caryocinèse de *Secale cereale* et sur une cause d'erreur dans la numération de ses chromosomes. Bull. Soc. Roy. Bot. Belgium 55: 186–89.

FERWERDA, F. P., 1948. Enkele waarnemingen over inteelt en heterosis bij rogge. Studiekring voor Plantenveredel. 3.: 226–29.

FERWERDA, F. P., 1951. Inteelt en heterosis bij rogge. Landbouwk. Tijdschr. 63: 319–30.

FETISSOV, A. I., 1939. Reduction division in the 16-chromosome rye. Compt. Rend. (Dokl.) Akad. Sci. URSS 25: 146–47.

FLORELL, V. H., 1931. A genetic study of wheat-rye hybrids and backcrosses. Journ. Agric. Res. 42: 315–39.

FRIMMEL, F., 1939. Beitrag zur Xenianfrage bei Roggen. Züchter II: 301–07.

FRIMMEL, F. and J. BARANEK, 1935. Beitrag zur Methodik der Roggenzüchtung und des Roggensaatgutbaues. Zschr. Pflanzenz. 20: 1–22.

FRUWIRTH, C., 1923. Roggen (*Secale cereale*). Handb. landw. Pflanzenz. 4: 200–48.

GAINES, E. F. and F. J. STEVENSON, 1922. Rye-wheat and wheat-rye hybrids. Journ. Hered. 13: 81–90.

GARBINI, S. E., 1950. (Behaviour of varieties of oats, barley and rye tested at Pergamino). Rept. 4th Meeting Perg. Expt. Sta. 231–34.

GASSNER, G. and E. NIEMANN, 1954. Symptome der Steinbranderkrankung (*Tilletia*) bei Weizen und Roggen. Phytopath. Zschr. 22: 288–300.

GATES, R. R., 1942. Nucleoli and related nuclear structures. Bot. Rev. 8: 337–409.

GAUL, H., 1953. Genomanalytischen Untersuchungen bei *Triticum* × *Agropyrum intermedium* unter Berücksichtigung von *Secale cereale* × *A. intermedium*. Zschr. ind. Abst. Vererb. L. 85: 505–46.

GAUL, H., 1954. Über meiotische Fragment- und Brückenbildung der Bastarde *Secale* und *Triticum* × *Agropyrum*. Chromosoma 6: 314–29.

GOFFART, H., 1951. Nematoden der Kulturpflanzen Europas. Parey, Berlin.

GOTOH, K., 1924. Über die Chromosomenzahl von *Secale cereale* L. Bot. Mag. Tokyo 38: 135–52.

GOTOH, K., 1932. Further investigations on the chromosome number of *Secale cereale* L. Jap. Journ. Genet. 7: 172-82.

GROSSHEIM, A. A., 1924. (A new variety of wild mountain rye in Transcaucasia). Bull. Appl. Bot. 13: 461–82.

HÅKANSSON, A., 1948. Behaviour of accessory rye chromosomes in the embryo sac. Hereditas 34: 35–59.

HÅKANSSON, A., 1957. Meiosis and pollen mitosis in rye plants with many accessory chromosomes. Hereditas 43: 603–19.

HÅKANSSON, A. and S. ELLERSTRÖM, 1950. Seed development after reciprocal crosses between diploid and tetraploid rye. Hereditas 36: 256–96.

HALL, O., 1954. Hybridization of wheat and rye after embryo transplantation. Hereditas 40: 453–58.

HASEGAWA, N., 1934. A cytological study on 8-chromosome rye. Cytologia 6: 68–77.

HAUPT, W., 1928. Die Schartigkeit des Winterroggens. Georgia 105: 672–73.

HECTOR, J., 1934. Introduction to Botany of Field Crops.

HERIBERT-NILSSON, N., 1913. Einige Beobachtungen über erbliche Variationen der Chlorophylleigenschaft bei den Getreidearten. Zschr. ind. Abst. Vererb. L. 9: 289–300.

HERIBERT-NILSSON, N., 1916. Populationanalysen und Erblichkeitsversuche über die Selbststerilität, Selbstfertilität und Sterilität bei dem Roggen. Zschr. Pflanzenz. 4: 1–44.

HERIBERT-NILSSON, N., 1917. Versuche über den Vizinismus des Roggens mit einem pflanzlichen Indikator. Zschr. Pflanzenz. 5: 89–114.

HERIBERT-NILSSON, N., 1937. Einige Prüfung der Wege und Theorien der Inzucht. Hereditas 39: 236–56.

HERIBERT-NILSSON, N., 1953. Über die Entstehung der Selbstfertilität beim Roggen. Hereditas 39: 65–74.

HILPERT, G., 1957. Effect of selection for meiotic behaviour in autotetraploid rye. Hereditas 43: 318–22.

HINTZER, H. M. R. and H. MIRANDA, 1954. Investigations on the quality of diploid and tetraploid rye for breadmaking. Cereal Chem. 31: 407–16.

HORNBURG, P., 1929. Untersuchungen über eine Roggenabnormalität. Zschr. Pflanzenz. 14: 509–12.

ISENBECK, K. and K. v. ROSENSTIEL, 1950. Die Züchtung des Weizens (Sonderausg. Handb. Pflanzenz. I. Aufl.).

JAIN, S. K., 1958. Fitting the negative binomial distribution to some data on asynaptic behaviour of chromosomes. Genetica 30 (in Press).

JAIN, S. K., 1959. Über das Vorkommen einer heteromorphischen Bivalenten in *Secale vavilovii*. Cytologia (in Press).

JENSEN, N. F. and G. C. KENT, 1952. Disease resistance from a wheat × rye cross. Journ. Hered. 43: 242.

JOST, L., 1907. Über die Selbststerilität einiger Blüten. Bot. Zeit. 65: 77–117.

JONES, J. W. and N. F. JENSEN, 1954. Behaviour of the hairy-neck character in wheat-rye hybrids. Agron. Journ. 46: 78–80.

KAGAWA, F. and Y. CHIZAKI, 1934. Cytological studies on the genus hybrids among *Triticum*, *Secale* and *Aegilops* and the species hybrids in *Aegilops*. Jap. Journ. Bot. 7: 1–32.

KAKHIDZE, N. J., 1939. (Meiosis in inbred rye). C.R. (Dokl.) Akad. Sci. URSS 25: 68–70.

KALT, B., 1916. Ein Beitrag zur Kenntnis chlorophylloser Getreidepflanzen. Zschr. Pflanzenz. 4: 143–50.

KARPECHENKO, G. D. and O. N. SOROKINA, 1929. The hybrids of *Aegilops triuncialis* with rye. Bull. App. Bot. 20: 563–84.

KARPETZAN, V. K., 1954. (Genetic analyses of a rye-wheat and wheat-rye hybrid). Agrobiologija 3: 67–80.

KATTERMANN, G., 1937. Chromosomenuntersuchungen bei halmbehaarten Stämmen aus Weizen-Roggen Bastardierung. Zschr. ind. Abst. Vererb. L. 73: 1–48.

KATTERMANN, G., 1938a. Das Verhalten des Chromosomes für Behaarung roggenbehaarter Nachkommen aus Weizenroggenbastardierung in neuen Kreuzungen mit Roggen und Weizen. Zschr. ind. Abst. Vererb. L. 74: 1–16.

KATTERMANN, G., 1938b. Über konstante halmbehaarte Stämme aus Weizenroggenbastardierung mit 2n=42 Chromosomen. Zschr. ind. Abst. Vererb. L. 74: 354–75.

KATTERMANN, G., 1939. Ein neuer Karyotyp bei Roggen. Chromosoma 1: 284–99.

KIHARA, H., 1924. Cytologische und genetische Studien bei wichtigen Getreidearten mit besonderer Rücksicht auf das Verhalten der Chromosomen und die Sterilität in den Bastarden. Mem. Coll. Sci. Kyoto B: I: 1–200.

KONDO, N., 1941. Chromosome doubling in *Secale, Haynaldia* and *Aegilops* by colchicine treatment. Jap. Journ. Genet. 17: 46–54.

KOO, F. K. S., 1958. Deleterious effects from interpollination of diploid and autotetraploid winter rye varieties. Agron. Journ. 50: 171–72.

KÖRNICKE, F., 1885. Handbuch des Getreidebaues. Bd. 1 u. 2. Parey, Berlin.

KOSTOFF, D., 1937. Interspecific hybrids in *Secale*. 1. *Secale cereale* × *S. ancestrale, S. cereale* × *S. vavilovii* and *S. ancestrale* × *vavilovii* hybrids. C.R. (Dokl.) Akad. Sci. URSS 14: 213–14.

KOSTOFF, D., 1939a. Frequency of polyembryony and chlorophyll deficiency in rye. C.R. (Dokl.) Akad. Sci. URSS 24: 479–82.

KOSTOFF, D., 1939b. Induction of polyploidy by pulp and disintegrating tissues from *Colchicum*. Nature 143: 287–88.

KOSTOFF, D., N. DOGADKENA and A. TRICHONOVA, 1935. Chromosome numbers of certain angiosperm plants. C.R. (Dokl.) Akad. Sci. URSS 3: 401–04.

KOTHOFF, P., 1942. Die Resistenz von Roggensorten gegen *Anguillulina (Ditylenchus) dipsaci*. Angew. Bot. 24: 79–99.

KRANZ, A. R., 1957. Populationsgenetische Untersuchungen am iranischen Primitivroggen. Zschr. Pflanzenz. 38: 101–46.

KRASNJUK, A. A., 1935. (The hybrid of *Secale cereale* × *Agropyron cristatum*). Social Grain Farming 5: 106–14.

KRASNJUK, A. A., 1936. (Some findings on the genetics of rye). Br. and Seedgr. 9: 50–53.

KRESS, H., 1938. (The correlation between growth observations and yield). Diss. Univ. Bonn. 61 pp.

LADA, P., 1933. (The genetics of brittle rye). Bull. Intern. Acad. Pol. Sci. Math. Nat. I: 183–93.

LAMM, R., 1936. Cytological studies on inbred rye. Hereditas 22: 217–40.

LAMM, R., 1944. Chromosome behaviour in a triploid rye plant. Hereditas 30: 137–44.

LANDES, M., 1939. The cause of self-sterility in rye. Amer. Journ. Bot. 26: 567–70.

LAUBE, H. A., 1956. Vergleichende Untersuchungen zur Entwicklungsphysiologie am Petkuser Normalstroh Roggen (2n) und Petkuser Tetreroggen (4n). Zschr. Pflanzenz. 36: 305–62.

LAUBE, W. and F. QUADT, 1956. Roggen (*Secale cereale* L.). Handbuch der Pflanzenz. 2. Aufl. II. Band. 35–102.

LAWRENCE, C. W., 1958. Genotypic control of chromosome behaviour in rye. VI. Selection for disjunction frequency. Heredity 12: 127–31.

LEDINGHAM, G. F. and W. P. THOMPSON, 1938. The cytogenetics of nonamphidiploid derivatives of wheat-rye hybrids. Cytologia 8: 377–97.

LEIGHTY, C. E. W. J. SANDO and J. W. TAYLOR, 1926. Intergeneric hybrids in *Aegilops*, *Triticum* and *Secale*. Journ. Agric. Res. 33: 101–41.

LEIGHTY, C. E. and J. W. TAYLOR, 1924. Hairy-neck wheat segregates from wheat-rye hybrids. Journ. Agric. Res. 28: 567–76.

LEIN, A., 1943a. Die Wirksamkeit von Kreuzbarkeitsgenen des Weizens in Kreuzungen von Roggen ♀ mit. Weizen ♂. Züchter 15: 1–3.

LEIN, A., 1943b. Die genetische Grundlage der Kreuzbarkeit zwischen Weizen und Roggen. Zschr. ind. Abst. Vererb. L. 81: 28–61.

LEISER, M., 1954. Die Bastardierung von Weizen und Roggen auf Grund experimenteller Untersuchungen unter besonderer Berücksichtigung der zytologischen Verhältnisse und deren Beziehungen zu aussern und innern Eigenschaften. Zschr. Pflanzenz. 33: 59–98.

LEITH, B. D., 1925. Sterility in rye. Journ. Amer. Soc. Agron. 17: 129–32.

LEITH, B. D. and H. L. SHANDS, 1938. Fertility as a factor in rye improvement. Journ. Amer. Soc. Agron. 30: 406–18.

LEKEZYNSKA, J. and J. WIONECK, 1954. (Conditions governing the formation of branched ears in rye). Acta agrobot. Warzawa 2: 103–08.

LEVAN, A., 1942. Studies on the meiotic mechanism of haploid rye. Hereditas 28: 177–211.

LEVAN, A., 1943. The pigment content of polyploid plants. Hereditas 29: 255–68.

LEVINE, M. N. and E. C. STAKMAN, 1923. Biologic specialization of *Puccinia graminis secalis*. Phytopath. 13: 35 (Abst.).

LEWITSKY, G. A., 1929. Investigations on the morphology of chromosomes. Proc. USSR Cong. Genet. Pl. and Anim. Breed., 2: 87–105.

LEWITSKY, G. A., 1931. The morphology of chromosomes. Bull. Appl. Bot. 27: 19–174.

LEWITSKY, G. A. A. N. MELNIKOV and N. N. TITOVA, 1932. (The cytology of the offspring of the 16-chromosome rye). Bull. Lab. Genet. 9: 89–96.

LIMA-DE-FARIA, A., 1948. B-chromosomes of rye at pachytene. Portug. Acta Biol. (A) 2: 167–74.

Lima-de-Faria, A., 1949. Genetics, origin and evolution of kinetochores. Hereditas 35: 422–44.

Lima-de-Faria, A., 1952a. The chromomere size gradient of the chromosomes of rye. Hereditas 38: 246–48.

Lima-de-Faria, A., 1952b. Chromomere analysis of the chromosome complement of rye. Chromosoma 5: 1–68.

Lima-de-Faria, A., 1955a. Structure and behaviour of a chromosome derivative with a deleted kinetochore. Chromosoma 7: 51–77.

Lima-de-Faria, A., 1955b. Structural differentiation of the kinetochore in rye and *Agapanthus*. Chromosoma 7: 78–89.

Lima-de-Faria, 1956. The role of the kinetochore in chromosome organization. Hereditas 42: 85–160.

Lima-de-Faria, A. and P. Sarvella, 1958. The organization of telomeres in species of *Solanum, Salvia, Scilla, Secale, Agapanthus* and *Ornithogalum*. Hereditas 44: 337–46.

Longley, A. E. and W. J. Sando, 1930. Nuclear divisions in the PMC's of *Triticum, Aegilops* and *Secale* and their hybrids. Journ. Agric. Res. 40: 683.

Love, H. H. and W. T. Craig, 1919. Fertile wheat-rye hybrids. Journ. Hered. 10: 195–207.

Löwenstein, J., 1951. Über die Befruchtungverhältnisse zwischen diploidem und tetraploidem Roggen. Zschr. Pflanzenz. 31: 104–33.

Lundqvist, A., 1947. On selfsterility and inbreeding effect of tetraploid rye. Hereditas 33: 570–71.

Lundqvist, A., 1953. Inbreeding in autotetraploid rye. Hereditas 39: 19–32.

Lundqvist, A., 1954. Studies on self-sterility in rye (*Secale cereale* L.). Hereditas 40: 278–94.

Lundqvist, A., 1956. Self-incompatibility in rye. I. Genetic control in the diploid. Hereditas 42: 293–348.

Lundqvist, A., 1958. Self-incompatibility in rye. III. Homozygosity for incompatibility factors in relation to viability and vegetative development. Hereditas 44: 174–188.

Lundqvist, A., 1958. Self-incompatibility in rye. IV. Factors related to self-seeding. Hereditas 44: 193–256.

Mains, E. B., 1926. Rye resistant to leaf rust, stem rust and powdery mildew. Journ. Agric. Res. 32: 201–21.

Mains, E. B. and C. E. Leighty, 1923. Resistance in rye to leaf rust, *Puccinia dispersa* Erikss. Journ. Agric. Res. 25: 243–52.

Mather, K. and R. Lamm, 1935. The negative correlation of chiasma frequencies. Hereditas 20: 65–70.

Matsuura, H., 1933. A bibliographical monograph on plant genetics. 1900–1929. Hokkaido. 2nd edition.

Mayer, H. K., 1944. Iets over inteelt-proefnemingen bij rogge. Studiekring Plantenveredel. Wageningen 44: 15–18.

McClintock, B., 1933. The association of nonhomologous parts of chromosomes in the midprophase of *Zea mays*. Zschr. Zellf. und Mikr. Anat. 19: 191–237.

MEISTER, G. K., 1928. Das Problem der Speziesbastardierung in Lichte der experimentellen Methode. Zschr. ind. Abst. Vererb. L. Suppl. 1094–1117.

MENGERSEN, F. G., 1950. Untersuchungen über die Ausnutzung von Inzucht und Heterosis in der Roggenzüchtung. DLG-Nachr. Pflanzenz. 115–33.

MENGERSEN, F. G., 1951. Die Wirkung der Inzucht auf verschiedene Merkmale beim Roggen. Zschr. Pflanzenz. 30: 218–48.

MENGERSEN, F. G. and W. SCHNELL, 1956. Untersuchungen zur Heterosis bei Roggen. Zschr. Pflanzenz. (cited after LAUBE and QUADT, 1956).

MORRISON, J. W., 1956. Chromosome behaviour and fertility of tetra Petkus rye. Canad. Journ. Agric. Sci. 36: 157–65.

MOTHES, K. and A. SILBER, 1952. Über die Vitalität des Mutterkorns. Forsch. und Fortsch. 28: 101.

MÜNTZING, A., 1936. The evolutionary significance of autopolyploidy. Hereditas 21: 263–378.

MÜNTZING, A., 1937a. Polyploidy from twin seedlings. Cytologia, Fujii Jub. Vol. 211–27.

MÜNTZING, A., 1937b. Note on a haploid rye plant. Hereditas 23: 401–04.

MÜNTZING, A., 1938. Note on heteroploid twin plants from eleven genera. Hereditas 24: 487–91.

MÜNTZING, A., 1939a. Studies on the properties and the ways of production of rye-wheat amphiploids. Hereditas 25: 387–430.

MÜNTZING, A., 1939b. Chromosomeanberrationen bei Pflanzen und ihre genetische Wirkung. Zschr. ind. Abst. Vererb. L. 76: 323–50.

MÜNTZING, A., 1943a. Double crosses of inbred rye. Bot. Notiser 1943 333–45.

MÜNTZING, A., 1943b. Aneuploidy and seed shrivelling in tetraploid rye. Hereditas 29: 65–75.

MÜNTZING, A., 1943c. Genetical effects of duplicated fragment chromosomes in rye. Hereditas 29: 91–112.

MÜNTZING, A., 1944. Cytological studies on extra-fragments chromosomes in rye. I. Isofragments produced by misdivision. Hereditas 30: 231–48.

MÜNTZING, A., 1945. Cytological studies of extra-fragment chromosomes in rye. II. Transmission and multiplication of standard fragments and isofragments. Hereditas 31: 457–77.

MÜNTZING, A., 1946a. Cytological studies of extra-fragment chromosomes in rye. III. The mechanism of nondisjunction at the pollen mitosis. Hereditas 32: 97–119.

MÜNTZING, A., 1946b. Sterility in rye populations. Hereditas 32: 521–49.

MÜNTZING, A., 1948a. Cytological studies of extra-fragment chromosomes in rye. V. A new fragment type arisen by deletion. Hereditas 34: 435–42.

MÜNTZING, A., 1949. Accessory chromosomes in *Secale* and *Poa*. Proc. 8th Intern. Cong. Genet. (Hereditas suppl.) 402–11.

MÜNTZING, A., 1950. Accessory chromosomes in rye populations from Turkey and Afghanistan. Hereditas 36: 507–09.

MÜNTZING, A., 1951a. Cytogenetic properties and practical value of tetraploid rye. Hereditas 37: 17–84.

MÜNTZING, A., 1951b. The meiotic pairing of isochromosomes in rye. Portug. Acta Biol. Ser. A. R. B. Goldschmidt: 831–60.

MÜNTZING, A., 1954a. Cytogenetics of accessory chromosomes (B chromosomes). Caryologia Suppl. 6: 282–301.

MÜNTZING, A., 1954b. An analysis of hybrid vigour in tetraploid rye. Hereditas 40: 265–77.

MÜNTZING, A., 1957. Frequency of accessory chromosomes in rye strains from Korea. Wheat Inf. Service 5: July, 1957.

MÜNTZING, A. and S. AKDIK, 1948a. The effect on cell size of accessory chromosomes in rye. Hereditas 34: 248–50.

MÜNTZING, A. and S. AKDIK, 1948b. Cytological disturbances in the first inbred generations of rye. Hereditas 34: 485–509.

MÜNTZING, A. and A. LIMA-DE-FARIA, 1949. Pachytene analysis of standard fragments and large isofragments in rye. Hereditas 35: 253–68.

MÜNTZING, A. and A. LIMA-DE-FARIA, 1952. Pachytene analysis of a deficient accessory chromosome in rye. Hereditas 38: 1–10.

MÜNTZING, A. and A. LIMA-DE-FARIA, 1953. Pairing and transmission of a small accessory iso-chromosome in rye. Chromosoma 6: 142–48.

MÜNTZING, A. and R. PRAKKEN. Chromosomal aberrations in rye populations. Hereditas 27: 273–308.

MÜNTZING, A. and E. RUNQUIST, 1939. Note on some colchicine-induced polyploids. Hereditas 25: 492–95.

NAKAJIMA, G., 1942. (Cytogenetical studies of triple hybrids from F_1 Triticum turgidum × Secale cereale and Triticum vulgalre. I. Number of somatic chromosomes and external characters). Proc. Imp. Acad. Tokyo 18: 100–06.

NAKAJIMA, G., 1948. (Karyogenetical investigations on the fertile F_1 plant between T. turgidum × Secale cereale). Proc. Crop. Soc. Japan, 16.

NAKAJIMA, G., 1950a. (Genetical and cytological studies in the breeding of amphidiploid types between Triticum and Secale. I. The external characters and chromosomes of the fertile F_1 T. turgidum (n = 14) × S. cereale (n = 7) and its F_2 progenies). Jap. Journ. Gen. 25: 139–48.

NAKAJIMA, G., 1950b. II. The external characters and chromosomes of the fertile F_1 T. compactum × S. cereale and its F_2 progenies). Jap. Journ. Genet. 25: 191–99.

NAKAJIMA, G., 1951. (Cytogenetical studies on intergeneric hybrids between Haynaldia and Secale. I. Morphology and meiosis in PMC's of an F_1 plant of H. villosa × S. cereale). La Kromosomo 9/10: 364–69.

NAKAJIMA, G , 1952. Cytological studies on intergeneric F§ hybrid between Triticum and Secale, with special reference to the number of bivalents in meiosis of PMC's. Cytologia 17: 144–55.

NAKAJIMA, G., 1953a. A cytological study on the intergeneric hybrid between T. sphaerococcum and S. cereale. Cytologia 18: 43–49.

NAKAJIMA, G., 1953b. (On the chromosomes of 3 species of genus Secale). Jap. Journ. Breed. 2: 201–04.

NAKAJIMA, G., 1954a. (Autotetraploid rye produced by the colchicine method). Jap. Journ. Breed. 4: 41–43.

NAKAJIMA, G., 1954b. (Cytogenetical studies of interspecific hybrids of *Secale*. I. The results of hybridization and the external morphology of the F_1 plants). Jap. Journ. Breed. 4: 132–34.

NAKAJIMA, G., 1954c. (A rye with 2n = 19 chromosomes). Jap. Journ. Breed. 4: 149–52.

NAKAJIMA, G., 1954d. Cytogenetical studies on the intergeneric F_1 hybrids between *Triticum vulgare* and three species of *Secale*. Jap. Journ. Bot. 14: 194–214.

NAKAJIMA, G., 1954c. Chromosomes of *Secale Kuprijanovii* Grossh. Bot. Mag. Tokyo 67: 69–72.

NAKAJIMA, G., 1955. Cytogenetic studies on *Triticum compactum* × *Secale cereale* F_1 hybrids. La kromosomo 22/24: 816–23.

NAKAJIMA, G., 1956. (Cytogenetical studies on interspecific hybrids of rye. II. Meiosis in pollen mother cells of F_1 between *Secale cereale* on one hand and *S. vavilovii*, *S. africanum* and *S. montanum* on the other). Jap. Journ. Breed. 6: 171–74.

NAKAJIMA, G., 1956b. (The chromosomes of *Secale fragile* and two varieties of *S. montanum*). La kromosomo 29: 1020–24.

NAKAO, M., 1911. Cytological studies on the nuclear divisions of PMC's of some cereals and their hybrids. J. Coll. Agric. Tohoku Imp. Univ. 4: 173–90.

NAVASHIN, M., 1934. Chromosome alterations caused by hybridization and their bearing upon certain general genetic problems. Cytologia 5: 169–203.

NEMEČ, B., 1910. Das Problem der Befruchtungsvorgänge und andere zytologische Fragen. (Cited after EMME, 1928).

NEUMANN-PELSHENKE, P., 1954. Brotgetreide und Brot. Parey, Berlin.

NICOLAISEN, W., 1932. Über quantitative Xenien bei Roggen und Erbsen. Zschr. Pflanzenz. 17: 265–76.

NOGGLE, G. R., 1947. A chemical study of diploid and tetraploid rye. Lloydia, Cincinn. 10: 19–37.

NORDENSKIÖLD, H., 1939. Studies of a haploid rye plant. Hereditas 25: 204–10.

NURNBERG-KRÜGER, U., 1947. Die Wirkung einer Bestaubungbeschränkung beim Roggen und ihre Erklärung. Züchter 17: 146–53.

NURNBERG-KRÜGER, U., 1951. Über die Answirkung des Plasmas auf Leistungsmerkmale beim Roggen. Züchter 21: 232–40.

OEHLER, E., 1938. Untersuchungen über die Behaarung des Halmes in Nachkommenschaften aus Weizen-Roggen-Kreuzungen. Zschr. Pflanzenz. 22: 417–51.

OINUMA, T., 1952. (Karyomorphology of cereals). Biol. Journ. Okayama Univ. I: 12–71.

OINUMA, T., 1953a. (Nuclear morphology of the cereals. II. On karyotype alteration in rye). Jap. Journ. Genet. 28: 28–34.

OINUMA, T., 1953b. (Karyomorphological studies on the origin of 8- and 9-chromosome rye). Jap. Journ. Genet. 28: 57–62.

O'MARA, J., 1940. Cytogenetic studies on *Triticale*. I. A method for determining the effects of individual *Secale* chromosomes on *Triticum*. Genetics 25: 401–08.

O'MARA, J., 1943. Meiosis in autotetraploid *Secale cereale*. Bot. Gaz. 104: 563–75.

O'MARA, J., 1948. Fertility in allopolyploids. Rec. Genet. Soc. Amer. 17: 52.

O'MARA, J., 1951. Cytogenetic studies on *Triticale*. II. The kinds of intergeneric chromosome addition. Cytologia 16: 225–32.

O'MARA, J., 1953. The cytogenetics of *Triticale*. Bot. Rev. 19: 587–605.

OSSENT, H. P., 1930. Perennierender Kulturroggen. Züchter 2: 221–27.

OSSENT, H. P., 1938. 10 Jahre Roggenzüchtung in Müncheberg. Züchter 10: 255–61.

ÖSTERGREN, G., 1947. Heterochromatic B-chromosomes in *Anthoxanthum*. Hereditas 33: 261–96.

ÖSTERGREN, G., and R. PRAKKEN, 1946. Behaviour on the spindle of the actively mobile chromosome ends of rye. Hereditas 32: 473–94.

PATHAK, G. N., 1940. Studies in the cytology of cereals. Journ. Benet. 39: 437–67.

PETERS, R., 1954. Vorselektion induzierter autopolyploider Gersten- und Roggen keimlinge nach der Wurzeldicke. Züchter 24: 128–31.

PETERSON, R. F., 1934. Improvement of rye through inbreeding. Sci. Agric. 14: 651–68.

PLAHN, R., 1927. Das Problem der Schartigkeit beim Roggen. Deutsch. landw. Pr.

PLARRE, W., 1953. Vergleichende Untersuchungen an diploidem und tetraploidem Roggen unter besonderer Berücksichtigung von Inzuchterscheinung und Fertilitätsstörungen. Kühn Archiv. 67: 398–99.

PLARRE, W., 1954. Vergleichende Untersuchungen an diploidem und tetraploidem Roggen. Zschr. Pflanzenz. 33: 303—53.

POPOFF, A., 1939. Untersuchungen über den Formenreichtum und die Schartigkeit des Roggens. Angew. Bot. 21: 325–56.

PRAKKEN, R., 1943. Studies of asynapsis in rye. Hereditas 29: 475–95.

PRAKKEN, R. and A. MÜNTZING, 1942. A meiotic peculiarity in rye simulating a terminal centromere. Hereditas 28: 441–82.

PRAKKEN, R. and M. S. SWAMINATHAN, 1951. Experience with the hydroxyquinoline smear method. Meded. Landb. Hoog. Wagen. 50: 137–40.

PRICE, S., 1955a. Induction of additional hybrid sterility in *Secale cereale* × *S. montanum* by irradiation of pollen. Science 121: 625–26.

PRICE, S., 1955b. Irradiation and interspecific hybridization in *Secale*. Genetics 40: 651–67.

PURVIS, O. N., 1939. Studies in vernalization of cereals. IV. The inheritance of the spring and winter habit in hybrids of Petkus rye. Ann. Bot. n.s. 3: 719–30.

PUTT, E. D., 1954. Cytogenetic studies in rye. Canad. Journ. Plant Sci. 34: 81–119.

QUINCKE, F. L., 1940. Interspecific and intergeneric crosses with *Hordeum*. Canad. Journ. Res., Sec. C. 18: 372–73.

REES, H., 1955a. Genotypic control of chromosome behaviour in rye. I. Inbred lines. Heredity 9: 93–116.

REES, H., 1955b. Heterosis in chromosome behaviour. Proc. Roy. Soc., Ser. B: 144: 150–59.

REES, H., 1957. Genotypic control of chromosome behaviour in rye. IV. The origin of new variation. Heredity 11: 185–94.

REES, H. and J. B. THOMPSON, 1955. Localisation of chromosome breakage at meiosis. Heredity 9: 399–407.

REES, H. and J. B. THOMPSON, 1956. Genotypic control of chromosome behaviour in rye. III. Chiasma frequency in homozygotes and heterozygotes. Heredity 10: 409–24.

REES, H. and J. B. THOMPSON, 1958. Genotypic control of chromosome behaviour in rye. V. The distribution pattern of chiasmata between pollen mother cells. Heredity 12: 101–11.

RILEY, R., 1956. The cytogenetics of the differences between some *Secale* species. Journ. Agric. Sci. 46: 377–83.

RILEY, R., 1956. Adding individual rye chromosomes to wheat. Wheat Inf. Service 5.

RILEY, R. and V. CHAPMAN, 1957. The comparison of wheat-rye and wheat-*Aegilops* amphidiploids. Journ. Agric. Sci. 49: 246–50.

RILEY, R. and V. CHAPMAN, 1958. The production and phenotypes of wheat-rye chromosome addition lines. Heredity 12: 301–15.

ROD, J. and F. VRZEVSKII, 1954. (Breeding value of a winter rye with ears branching as a result of improved nutrient supply). Za. Social Setjsk. Nauk. Praha. Ser. A. 111–128.

ROEMER, TH., 1939. Handbuch der Pflanzenzüchtung, 2. Roggen (*Secale cereale* L.). Parey, Berlin. Pp. 34–74.

ROSHEVITZ, R. Y., 1948. (A monograph of the wild, weedy and cultivated species of rye). Acta Inst. Bot. Nom. V. L. Komarovii, Acad. Sci. URSS ser. I, Fl. et Supp. 6: 105–163. (English Translation by Dr. G. L. Stebbins).

RÜMKER, K., 1911. Etude sur le coloris des grains chez le seigle. IVe Cong. Génét. Paris: 332–35.

RÜMKER, K., 1912. Neue Ergebnisse meiner Züchtungsstudien auf dem Versuchfelde in Rosenthal. Zschr. Landw. 263–65.

SAKAMURA, T., 1918. Kurze Mitteilung über die Chromosomenzahlen und des Verwandtschaftverhältnisse der *Triticum*-Arten. Bot. Mag. Tokyo 32:151–54.

SANCHEZ-MONGE, E., 1956. (Studies on 42-chromosome *Triticale*. I. The production of the amphidiploids). Ann. Estac. Expt. de Aula Dei. 4: 191–207.

SCHEIBE, A., 1935. Die Verbreitung von Unkrautroggen und Taumalloch in Anatolien. Angew. Bot. 17: 1–22.

SCHIEMANN, E., 1932. Enstehung der Kulturpflanzen. Handb. Vererbungswiss. 3: 1–377.

SCHIEMANN, E., 1948. Weizen, Roggen, Gerste. Systematik, Geschichte, Verwendung. Fischer, Jena.

SCHIEMANN, E., 1949. Die neue Nomenklatur der Getreidearten. Züchter 19: 322–25.

SCHIEMANN, E. and U. NURNBERG-KRÜGER, 1952. Neue Untersuchungen an *Secale africanum* Stapf. Die Naturwiss. 6: 136–37.

SCHIEMANN, E. and H. G. SCHWEICKERDT, 1950. Neue Untersuchungen an *Secale africanum* Stapf. Bot. Jahrb. 75: 196–205.

SCHILDT, R. and E. ÅKERBERG, 1951. Studier over tetraploid och diploid rag vid Ultunafilialen. Sver. Utsadesfören. Tidskr. 61: 254–68.

SCHMUCK, A. and D. KOSTOFF, 1939. Brome-acenaphthene and brome-naptha-line as agents inducing chromosome doubling in rye and wheat. C.R. (Dokl.) Akad. Sci. URSS 23: 263.

SCHNEIDER, R., 1954. Der gegenwärtige Stand der Weizen-Roggen Bastardie-rung. Zschr. Pflanzenz. 5: 44–48.

SEARS, E. R., 1956. Weizen (*Triticum* L.). I. The systematics, cytology and genetics of wheat. Handb. der Pflanzenzücht. 9. Lief. Band II: 164–187.

SENGBUSCH, R., 1940a. Polyploider Roggen. Züchter 12: 185–89.

SENGBUSCH, R., 1940b. Pärchenzüchtung unter Ausschaltung von Inzucht-schäden. Forschungsdienst 10: 545–49.

SENGBUSCH, R., 1941. Polyploide Kulturpflanzen. (Roggen, Hafer, Stoppel-rüben, Kohlrüben und Radieschen). Züchter 13: 132–34.

SHMARGON, E. N., 1938a. New data on the morphology of rye chromosomes. C.R. (Dokl.) Akad. Sci. URSS 20: 43–45.

SHMARGON, E. N., 1938b. Analysis of the chromomere structure of mitotic chromosomes in rye. C.R. (Dokl.) Akad. Sci. URSS 21: 259–61.

SHMARGON, E. N., 1939. Chromomere structure of the chromosome set of rye. C.R. (Dokl.) Akad. Sci. URSS 23: 267–99.

SIRKS, M. J., 1929. Über einen Fall vererbbarer Lichtempfinlichkeit des Chloro-phylls beim Roggen (*Secale cereale*). Genetica II: 375–87.

SMAGIN, G. D., 1940. (An experiment on breeding double-eared rye). Jarovi-zacija 6: 105.

SMITH, D. C., 1942. Intergeneric hybridization of cereals and other grasses. Journ. Agric. Res. 64: 33–47.

SMITH, D. C., 1943. Relation of polyploidy to heat and X-ray effects in the cereals. Journ. Hered. 34: 131–34.

STEBBINS, G. L., 1949. The evolutionary significance of natural and artificial polyploids in the family *Gramineae*. Proc. 8th Intern. Congr. Genet. 461–85.

STEBBINS, G. L., 1950. Variation and Evolution in Plants. New York, U.P. Columbia 643 pp.

STEBBINS, G. L., 1956. Taxonomy and the evolution of genera, with special reference to the family *Gramineae*. Evolution 10: 235–45.

STEBBINS, C. L., 1958. The inviability, weakness and sterility of interspecific hybrids. Adv. Genet. 9: 147–215.

STEBBINS, G. L. and F. T. PUN, 1953. Artificial hybrids in the tribe Hordeae. IV. Chromosome pairing in *Secale cereale* × *Agropyron intermedium* and the problem of genome homologies in the Triticineae. Genetics 38: 600–08.

STEBBINS, G. L. and L. H. SNYDER, 1956. IX. Hybrids between Western and Eastern North American species. Amer. Journ. Bot. 43: 305–12.

STEGLEICH, L. and H. PIPER, 1922. Vererbungs- und Züchtungsversuche mit Roggen. Fühlings landw. Zbg. 71: 201–22.

STOLZE, K., 1925. Die Chromosomenzahlen der hauptsächlichsten Getreide-arten nebst allgemeinen Betrachtungen über Chromosomenzahl und Chromosomengrösse im Pflanzenreich. Bibliotheca Genet. 8: 8–71.

STUTZ, H. C., 1957. A cytogenetic analysis of the hybrid *Secale cereale* L. ×
S. montanum Guss. and its progeny. Genetics 42: 199–221.

STUTZ, H. C., 1958. A new macromutation in rye. Proc. Utah Acad. Sci. 34:
59–60.

SWANSON, C. R., 1957. Cytology and cytogenetics. Prentice Hall: 596 pp.

SYBENGA, J., 1958. Inbreeding effects in rye. Zeits. f. Vererbungslehre 89: 338–
54.

TAKAGI, F., 1935. Karyogenetical studies on rye. I. A trisomic plant. Cytologia
6: 496–501.

TAYLOR, J. W., 1934. Irregularities in the inheritance of the hairy-neck character transposed from *Secale* to *Triticum*. Journ. Agric. Res. 48: 603–17.

TAYLOR, J. W. and K. S. QUISENBERRY, 1935. Inheritance of rye crossability
in wheat hybrids. Journ. Amer. Soc. Agron. 27: 149–53.

THOMPSON, J. B., 1956. Genotypic control of chromosome behaviour in rye.
II. Disjunction at meiosis in interchange heterozygotes. Heredity 10:
99–108.

THOMPSON, J. B. and H. REES, 1956. Selection for heterozygotes during inbreeding. Nature 177: 385–86.

THOMPSON, W. P., 1922. Lethal factors in cereals. West. Canad. Soc. Agr. Proc.
3: 53–59.

THOMPSON, W. P., 1939. The frequency of fertilization and the nature of embryo
and endosperm development in intergeneric crosses in cereals. Proc. 7th
Intern. Cong. Genet. (Abstract).

THOMPSON, W. P., 1940. The causes of hybrid sterility and incompatibility.
Trans. Roy. Soc. Canada 34: 1–3.

THOMPSON, W. P. and D. JOHNSTON, 1945. The cause of incompatibility between barley and rye. Canad. Journ. Res. 23: 1–15.

THUMANIAN, M. G., 1938. Perennial semi-cultivated rye in Armenia. Sovetsk.
Bot. 6: 100–02.

TJIO, H. and A. LEVAN, 1950. The use of oxyquinoline in chromosome analysis.
Ann. Est. Aula Dei. 2: 21–64.

TJIO, H. and E. SANCHEZ-MONGE, 1954. (Spanish tetraploid ryes). Agric.
Madrid 22: 138–40.

TOTU, T., 1950. On the crossability between wheat and rye. Jap. Journ. Genet.
25: 90–95.

TREBOUX, O., 1925. Beobachtungen über Vererbung von Körnfarbe und Antho-
cyan beim Roggen. Zschr. Pflanzenz. 10: 288–91.

TSCHERMAK, E., 1906. Über Züchtung neuer Getreidearten mit künstlicher
Kreuzung. II. Mitteilung Kreuzungsstudien am Roggen. Zschr. Landw.
Vers. Oesterr. I: 1–45.

TSCHERMAK, E., 1913. Über seltene Getreidebastarde. Beitr. Pflanzenz. 3:
49–61.

TSCHERMAK, E., 1927. Über seltene Getreide- und Rübenbastarde. Zschr. ind.
Abst. Vererb. L. 2: 1495–98.

ÜLRICH, K., 1902. Die Bestäubung und Befruchtung des Roggens. Halle 1–62.

VASILIEV, B. L., 1940. (Wheat-rye hybrids. II. Genetic analysis of crossability of rye with various species of wheat). C.R. (Dokl.) Akad. Sci. URSS 27: 598–600.

VAVILOV, N. I., 1917. On the origin of cultivated rye. Bull. Appl. Bot. 10: 561–90.

VAVILOV, N. I., 1925. Studies on the origin of cultivated plants. Bull. Appl. Bot. 16: 1–248.

VAVILOV, N. I., 1928. Geographische Genzentren unserer Kulturpflanzen. 5th Intern. Cong. Genet. 342–69.

VERUSHKINE, S. and A. SHACHURDINE, 1933. Hybrids between wheat and couchgrass. Journ. Hered. 24: 329–35.

VILLAX, E. and M. MOTA, 1953. Behaviour of a *Triticum* × *Secale* hybrid under the action of colchicine. Nature 172: 412–13.

VRESKY, F., 1955. (The breeding value of branched ears in rye). Sborn. ecl. Acad. Za. 26: 371–86.

WARMBRUNN, K., 1952. Untersuchungen über den Zwergsteinbrand. Phytopath. Zschr. 19: 441–82.

WELLENSIEK, S. J., 1945. Methoden voor het kweken van aaltjesresistente rogge en enkele hieruit voortvloeiende consequenties voor de roggeveredeling in het algemeen. Studiekring v. Planten. Wagen. 45: 35–37.

WELLENSIEK, S. J., 1947. Rational methods for breeding crossfertilizers. Meded. Landb. Hogesch. 48: 227–62.

WELLENSIEK, S. J., 1948. Vegetatieve vermeerdering bij de veredeling, speciaal van groentegewassen. Meded. Inst. Veredel. Tuinbouw. 8: 57–71.

YAKUWA, K., 1944. (On the behaviour of supernumerary chromosomes of *Secale cereale* L.). Jap. Journ. Genet. 20: 72–73.

ZALENSKY, V. R. and A. V. DOROSHENKO, 1925. Zytologische Untersuchungen bei Weizen-roggenbastarden. Bull. Appl. Bot. 14: 185–210.

ZHUKOVSKY, P. M., 1928. (A wild growing form of rye in Anatolia). Bull. Appl. Bot. 19: 49–58.

ZHUKOVSKY, P. M., 1944. (Studies on hybridization and immunity of plants). K. A. Timiriasoff Acad. Agric. Moscow 6: 48–95.

ZIMMERMANN, K., 1951. Zwillingsauslese als Möglichkeit zur Züchtung von Fremdbefruchtern. Züchter 21: 253–55.